# Handbook o
# Fluids

Supradip Ghosh

# Handbook of Intravenous Fluids

Springer

Supradip Ghosh
Department of Critical Care Medicine
Fortis Escorts Hospital
Faridabad, Haryana, India

ISBN 978-981-19-0499-8 ISBN 978-981-19-0500-1 (eBook)
https://doi.org/10.1007/978-981-19-0500-1



This Springer imprint is published by the registered company Springer Nature Singapore Pte Ltd.
The registered company address is: 152 Beach Road, #21-01/04 Gateway East, Singapore 189721, Singapore

# Foreword

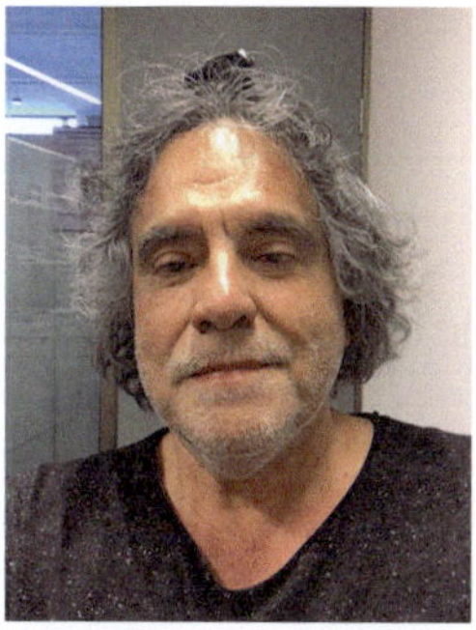

I've known rivers: I've known rivers ancient as the world and older than the flow of human blood in human veins.—Langston Hughes

When I was a child, we lived for some years in a city surrounded by three rivers. After endless and joyful walks along the shore with my parents, I grew up loving rivers. From the elegant Seine to the turbulent and wild Patagonian rivers, I recognize that most of the more poetic moments of my life have been experienced just sitting there at the shore of a river, simply fascinated by its continuous flow to distant and mysterious lakes or oceans.

As an intensivist, I always thought of fluid resuscitation as a metaphor of a river stream entering your veins with controlled intensity, always oscillating between the risks of insufficient flow or the inverse of massive flooding. Again, the old aphorism of "flow is life, and life is flow." In this sense, fluid therapy is the key of intensive care.

These thoughts and memories came to me after reading this wonderful gift by Dr. Supradip Ghosh. As a poet, I always believed that a medical book should be more than a classic, informative but eventually boring scholar text. Indeed, to build up a masterpiece is far more challenging. It must be holistic capturing pieces of strong background physiology but mixed up with clinical implications and bathed with accurate supporting evidence. It should be designed at to maintain the interest and rhythm of reading with an agile but sober design. It should have the wisdom to explain complex concepts with simple terms and lucid diagrams. It may also circle around recognizable clinical cases and problems, and bring solutions based on applied science and physiology, but expressed as simple recommendations.

Doubtlessly, this book is a masterpiece and it has been a long time since I didn't have on my hands a brilliant piece like this. A MUST read for any intensivist, or any physician, nurse, resident, or student dealing with acutely ill patients, whatever age or experience. But it is much more than that. Again, as a poet, I see here the best mixture or cocktail, the fusion between science and art! Moreover, I perceive passion, endless hours working in every delicate detail, but also love. Love for teaching, love for physiology, love for critical care, love for humanity!

And for all of this, I thank Dr. Supradip Ghosh for teaching us with this brilliant book on how to best manage the river of intensive care, fluid therapy.

Glenn Hernández

Intensive Care Medicine,
ANDROMEDA-SHOCK
Project
Pontificia Universidad
Católica de Chile
Santiago, Chile

# Foreword

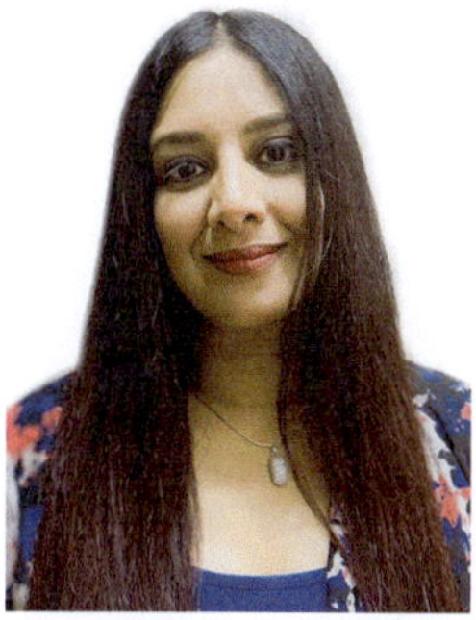

Patients may require fluid therapy to prevent or correct problems with their fluid or electrolyte status. Deciding on the optimal amount and composition of fluids to be administered and the best rate at which to give them can be a challenging task. These decisions require a good understanding of the physiology, clinical condition of the patient, and the types of fluid available.

It gives me immense pleasure to write a foreword for the *Handbook of Intravenous Fluid* written by Dr. Supradip Ghosh, an expert in the field of fluid management. Dr. Ghosh is the Director and Head of the Department of Critical Care Medicine at the Fortis-Escorts Hospital, Faridabad, India and the founder of the *Fluid Academy of India.*

The *Handbook of Intravenous Fluid* is an evidence-based ready to use pocket reference for intravenous fluid therapy. The author has covered most aspects of intravenous fluid therapy from physiology to the types of fluid and bedside clinical management. Important clinical trials in the field are summarized in relevant chapters. The author provides a succinct and practical format for each chapter using simple language with flowcharts, boxes, tables, and figures making it very useful for students. Each chapter starts with a case scenario followed by an introduction focusing on the learning objectives and finishing with the take-home message and recommendation.

This book will certainly be useful to clinicians dealing with acutely ill patients including (but not limited to) intensivists, emergency physicians, anesthesiologists, internists, other physicians and surgeons, especially for those practicing in developing countries.

Department of Anaesthesiology and Critical Care
Tata Memorial Hospital,
Mumbai, India

Sheila Nainan Myatra

# Preface

The prescription of intravenous fluid is almost a ubiquitous practice in acute care medicine. But a clear understanding of the subject is perhaps still lacking among practitioners, starting from basic questions like "why am I prescribing fluid to my patient" or "why a particular fluid" to practical issues like "how do I transcribe my thought process of intravenous fluid prescription in the case note" or "when shall I switch from intravenous to oral fluid." As a student of acute care medicine, as well as an educator, I felt the necessity of a ready to use evidence-based pocket reference for intravenous fluid prescription, covering various aspects in the field from physiology to bedside clinical management.

With this title "Handbook of Intravenous Fluids," I have tried to give a shape to my idea. The book opens up with review of basic physiology: rationale behind fluid therapy and physiological adaptations of human body to maintain homeostasis of different fluid compartments, internal and external balance. Heart–Lung Interaction being the central theme behind the concept of fluid responsiveness, I felt it necessary to have a dedicated chapter on the subject. The Chapter on acid–base physiology introduces readers to the concept provided by Peter Stewart, integrating changes in electrolyte composition of the body fluids to acid–base homeostasis, essential to understand effects of various commercially available intravenous fluid solutions on pH. The second section is dedicated to different commercially available intravenous fluid preparations. Apart from describing their composition, this section provides with up-to-date evidence behind their clinical use, helping readers to choose the right fluid for right clinical circumstances. Understanding concepts of fluid responsiveness and fluid challenge is essential for rational fluid prescription, especially in resuscitation scenarios. Section three of the book deals with these important areas of rational fluid therapy. Section three also introduces the reader to different phases of fluid resuscitation and also to the concept of de-resuscitation. The Fourth section provides readers with detail account of fluid prescription in common clinical scenarios: septic shock, hemorrhagic shock, diarrheal illnesses, burn, peri-operative period, and in diabetic ketoacidosis. As sodium homeostasis is closely related to overall fluid balance of the body, a chapter is dedicated to sodium disorder. Finally, in the last section, an attempt is made to integrate concepts provided in the book and provide readers with an approach to write an appropriate fluid prescription.

Taking advantage of being the sole author of the book, I attempted to maintain similar pattern throughout the book. Each chapter starts with a case scenario followed by an introduction focusing on the learning objectives and each chapter is completed with "take home messages" and important (but not a long list) of references. Visual elements such as flowcharts, boxes, tables, and figures are included in each chapter for easier understanding of the subject. In the era of "evidence-based medicine," important clinical trials in the field are summarized in relevant chapters, especially keeping in mind the need of students and fellows.

I hope this book will be useful for all clinicians dealing with acutely ill patients including (but not limited to) intensivists, emergency physicians, anesthesiologists, internists, other physicians and surgeons.

Best regards

Faridabad, India Supradip Ghosh

# Acknowledgement

Thank you, dear GOD, for being there with me and for helping me in preparing the manuscript.

This book might never have seen the light of the day without the enthusiastic support of my best friend and my soulmate, Dr. Sonali Ghosh. She has always been the greatest support through my thick and thin, from painstakingly going through each and every chapter of the manuscript for the first time and several times thereafter, to providing emotional and moral support when I was confused about the future of the project. Thank you, my love, for being there for me all the time, for believing in my ability. I love you.

What am I today is because of my parents Late Shri Manjugopal Ghosh and Mrs. Maya Ghosh. Thank you, "Ma" and "Baba," for being there for me. I thank my elder brother Mr. Jaydip Ghosh, members of my extended family, and my teachers for being with me and helping me in my life journey. I would also like to thank my son (no longer a boy but still not an adult officially), Rudraksha for bearing with me, during my long hours in reading and on MacBook, eating away his precious time with his parents. My special thanks to my closest friends, Dr. Anupam Kulshreshtha and Dr. Atul Sule for their constant support in difficult times.

I would also like to acknowledge contribution of my younger colleagues in the department and students, who have always been my inspiration for teaching, acquisition of new knowledge and acquiring new skills. I would especially like to thank my student Dr. Garima Arora for going through some of my initial chapters and for providing me with her perspective from a student's point of view. I appreciate efforts of all my colleagues from past and present for their help in shaping my career.

My heartfelt appreciation goes to everyone in Springer Nature who were involved in editing and publication of the manuscript.

# Contents

# About the Author

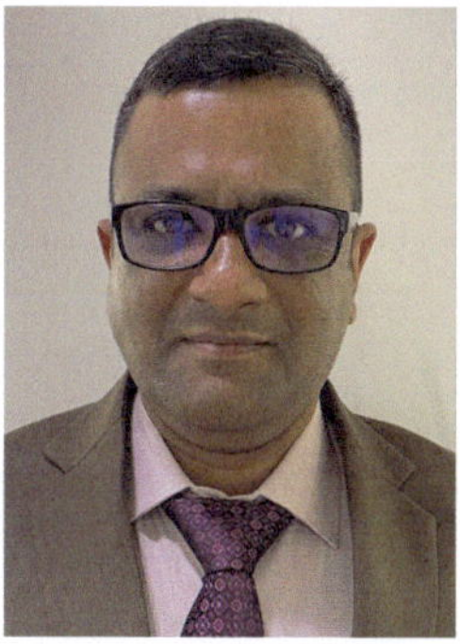

**Supradip Ghosh, DNB (Int Med), MRCP (UK), EDIC** is an intensive care physician with a passion for teaching. His areas of interest include rational management of intravenous fluid and resuscitation of acutely ill patients. With an aim to spread awareness about the rational use of intravenous fluid and to promote research in this field, he established the non-profit organisation "Fluid Academy of India" and the academy was registered under Indian law in January 2018. Under the Academy's banner Dr Ghosh has organised several conferences and workshops on fluid therapy in critically ill patients. He is currently working as the Director and Head, Department of Critical Care Medicine at Fortis-Escorts Hospital, Faridabad, India. Apart from being a regular faculty for all major critical care conferences conducted India, Dr Ghosh also have several peer-reviewed publications including book chapters and journal articles in national and international journals to his credit. He is also a recognised teacher and examiner for various critical care courses conducted in India. In recognition of his contribution in the field of Critical Care Medicine, he was awarded with prestigious "Fellow of Indian College of Critical Care Medicine (FICCM)" by the Indian Society of Critical Care Medicine in the year 2019.

# Part I
# Review of Physiology

# Chapter 1
# Guytonian Model of Circulation

## 1.1 Case Scenario

Mrs. RJ, an 84-year-old lady with a history of long-standing diabetes mellitus, hypertension and diabetic nephropathy presented to the emergency department with 2-days history of fever and burning micturition. Family noticed her to be confused since morning and decided to bring her to the hospital. Her regular medications include Metformin, Ramipril, Bisoprolol and low-dose Aspirin. On examination, she is drowsy but arousable. Her extremities are cold to touch with mottling seen on both thighs. She has a heart rate of 66/min and blood pressure of 70 mmHg systolic. Systemic examination findings are unremarkable except for tenderness on deep palpation of the right flank. Keeping in mind the possible diagnosis of pyelonephritis (right), urosepsis and septic shock in an elderly lady with diabetes, ED Physician decided to infuse 1000 ml of Ringer's Lactate over the next 30 min.



S. Ghosh, *Handbook of Intravenous Fluids*,
https://doi.org/10.1007/978-981-19-0500-1_1

### *1.1.1 How Does a Rapid Fluid Bolus Expected to Improve Systemic Perfusion?*

While managing a patient with circulatory shock, arguably the first thing that comes in mind, is rapid intravenous fluid bolus. Fluid bolus is infused with a hope of increasing cardiac output and ultimately to improve tissue perfusion. Our current understanding of the impact of fluid bolus on circulation is primarily based on the Guytonian model of circulatory dynamics. In this chapter, we shall reappraise the Guytonian physiology and possible effects of intravenous fluid on circulation.

## 1.2 Concept of Mean Systemic Pressure

- Bayliss and Starling coined the term **Mean Circulatory Filling Pressure** ($P_{mcf}$) as the average pressure throughout the circulation during circulatory arrest (e.g. immediately after administration of cardioplegia) [1].
  - A closely related and more widely used term is **Mean Systemic Pressure** ($P_{ms}$) defined as the equilibrium pressure only in the systemic circulation in the absence of any flow, ignoring the heart and pulmonary circulation (e.g. by clamping the aorta and venae cavae).
  - If we consider the whole circulatory system as pipelines, $P_{ms}$ can be seen as the elastic recoil potential stored in the walls of the pipeline.
- Elastic recoil potential is determined by the volume of blood that stretches these pipelines beyond maintaining their normal shape, also termed "**Stressed Volume**".
  - Remaining volume of blood that only maintains the shape of pipelines and does not contribute to elastic recoil potential is known as "**Unstressed Volume**".

- Normally only 30% of the blood volume (mostly stored in venous side of the circulation) contributes to the stressed volume.
  - "Stressed volume" and $P_{ms}$ can be increased either by increasing circulatory volume (e.g. by fluid loading) or by decreasing venous capacitance (e.g. by vasopressor infusion that converts unstressed volume to stressed volume).

## 1.3 Gradient to Venous Return

- Flow from peripheral circulation back to heart, otherwise known as **Venous Return** (VR), is directly proportional to the gradient (termed **Venous Return Gradient**) between $P_{ms}$ (the upstream pressure) and right atrial pressure (RAP, the downstream pressure) and inversely proportional to the resistance to venous return (or RVR).
  - This concept is based on Hagen–Poiseuille's law, conceptualized originally to understand the laminar flow of fluid through non-compressible pipes of constant proportion.
  - The concept can be described mathematically as:

$$VR = \frac{\left(P_{ms} - RAP\right)}{RVR}$$

(VR = Venous return, $P_{ms}$ = Mean systemic pressure, RAP = Right atrial pressure, RVR = Resistance to venous return)

- In physiological state, with constant blood volume and near-constant $P_{ms}$, the two most important factors that determine venous return are: right atrial pressure (RAP, the downstream pressure) and resistance to venous return (RVR).

- RVR and venous capacitance in turn is determined by local factors. For example, during states of high oxygen demand at the organ level, overall RVR is decreased because of the local release of vasodilator substances.
- Cardiac activity keeps the RAP closer to 0 mmHg, by constantly pumping out whatever blood volume coming back to it and helps in maintaining the gradient to venous return.

## 1.4 Venous Return Curve

- From their experiment on anaesthetized dogs, Guyton and colleagues demonstrated the effects of varying RAP (from very high positive to very low negative) on venous return [2]. They graphically represented their findings with RAP plotted on the *X*-axis and venous return on the *Y*-axis, what is now known as **Venous Return Curve**.
- Figure 1.1 shows a series of venous return curves.
  - On inspection of the left curve, one can appreciate that on progressive lowering of RAP, venous return increases until a point beyond which it remains in plateau state.

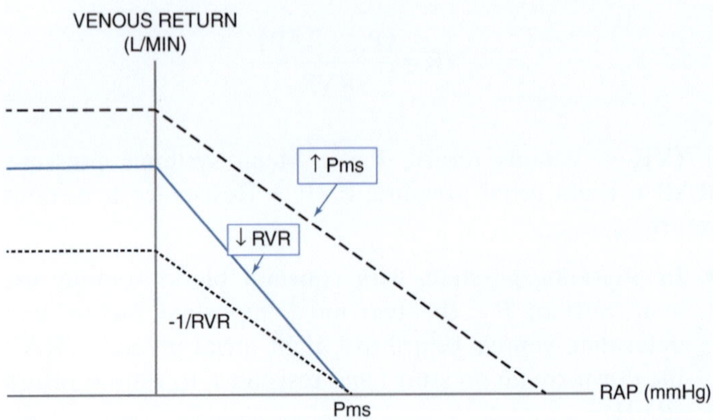


FIGURE 1.1 Venous return curves

This is because of the collapse of venae cavae at the thoracic inlet when the RAP value falls below surrounding pressure.
- Value of RAP at which the VR curve reaches the plateau is termed **Critical Pressure** ($P_{crit}$).

- In the intersection of venous return curve with the *X*-axis, $P_{ms}$ and RAP equalize, and (in theory only) venous return becomes zero.
  - In fact, this is one of the ways by which $P_{ms}$ can actually be measured (see Box 1.2 below)!
- The slope of the curve is related to −1/RVR, i.e. with a decrease in RVR, venous return curve is shifted clockwise (as can be seen in the middle curve of Fig. 1.1), increasing the Venous Return and vice versa.
- With an increase in $P_{ms}$, the venous return curve is shifted towards the right, resulting in an increase in VR (as can be seen in the right curve of Fig. 1.1).

## 1.5 Cardiac Function Curve

- Amount of blood ejected by the ventricle in a single cardiac cycle, also known as **Stroke Volume** (SV), is determined by three independent factors.
  - **Preload** defined as the length of the individual sarcomere at the end of ventricular filling (or at end-diastole), which in turn is determined by the end-diastolic volume. Ventricular intramural pressure at the end of diastole can be taken as a surrogate of ventricular preload.
  - **Afterload** defined as the load ventricle faces during ejection of blood or the transmural pressure at the root of aorta (for left ventricle) or root of pulmonary trunk (for right ventricle).
  - **Contractility** that may be defined as the elastance of ventricles, an intrinsic property of myocardial fibres.

- Amount of blood ejected by the ventricle in 1 min is known as "**Cardiac Output**" (CO).

$$CO = SV \times HR$$

  (HR, heart rate)

- Ventricles eject whatever volume of blood returned to their corresponding atria.
  - This was demonstrated by Patterson and Starling in their experiment on anaesthetized dogs [3].
  - They also noticed that with an increasing return of blood into the right atrium, there was only a slow increase in RAP. But beyond certain limit, there is an abrupt rise in RAP limiting further return of blood to the right atrium.
  - They graphically displayed their findings with return of blood to the right atrium (i.e. venous return) on the *X*-axis and RAP shown on the *Y*-axis (original "**Starling Curve**") [3].

- More than half a century after the original description of Starling curve, Guyton flipped the curve to describe his now-famous "**Cardiac Function Curve**".
  - With this change, Guyton showed the RAP on *X*-axis and cardiac output (in place of venous return) on *Y*-axis [4]. Guyton's idea was to integrate the return function and pump function of the heart, to develop an overall concept of circulation. This concept will be discussed further in later section.
  - This modified relationship between RAP and Cardiac Output ("**Cardiac Function Curve**"), also known today as **Frank–Starling Curve**, is shown in Fig. 1.2.

- However, cardiac function curve is not a single curve, but a series of curves. Shape of these curves depends on intrinsic cardiac contractility and ventricular afterload of a given patient.

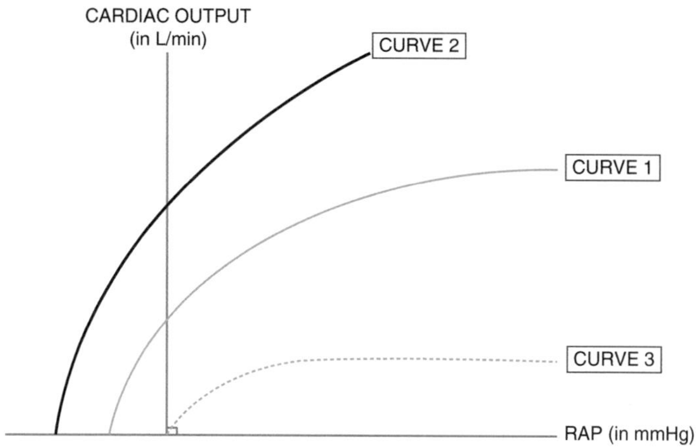


FIGURE 1.2 Cardiac function curves

– As can be seen in Curve 1 of Fig. 1.2, cardiac output reaches a plateau beyond a certain value of RAP (an unlikely situation practically!).
– With a decrease in afterload or an increase in intrinsic contractility, cardiac function curve is shifted upward and towards the left (Curve 2 in Fig. 1.2).
– In contrast, any increase in afterload or decrease in contractility shift the curve towards the right and downward (Curve 3 in Fig. 1.2).

## 1.6 Integrating the Return Function with Cardiac Function

• In a steady state, VR and CO must be equal (as confirmed in Starling experiments). Moreover, as both the venous return curve and cardiac function curve use RAP on *X*-axis, these two curves can be superimposed (that is what Guyton did!) [4].

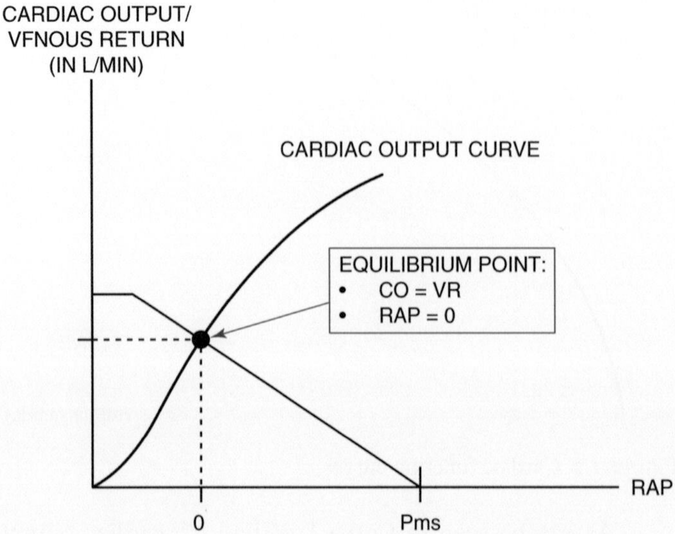


FIGURE 1.3 Integrated venous return and cardiac function curve

- As seen in Fig. 1.3, at the intersection of these two curves (also known as "**Equilibrium Point**"), VR is equal to CO.
- However, different clinical scenarios can change the equilibrium point (and thus cardiac output). These are discussed further in the next section.

## 1.7 Fluid Bolus, Vasopressors and Equilibrium Point

- Figure 1.4 graphically displays the overall effects of fluid bolus and vasoactive drugs on the cardiovascular system.
- **Effect of Fluid Bolus:** Rapid fluid bolus can increase the $P_{ms}$ by increasing stressed volume (as explained earlier) provided there is no profound vasoplegia or extreme capillary leak. This increase in $P_{ms}$ shifts the VR curve towards the right producing a new equilibrium point.

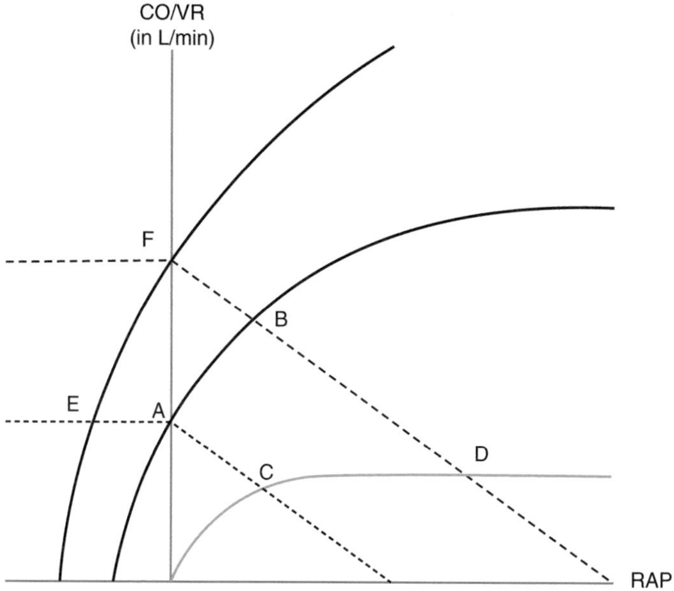


FIGURE 1.4 Effects of fluid bolus and vasoactive drugs on integrated cardiac function and venous return curves

- As shown in Fig. 1.4, shift of the venous return curve towards the right also shifts the equilibrium point from point A to point B with a corresponding increase in cardiac output. This increase in cardiac output is only possible if the equilibrium point is in the steep part of the cardiac function curve (so-called "**Permissive Heart**").
- Other minor mechanisms by which fluid bolus can increase the cardiac output are:

  a. By reducing the resistance to venous return and shifting the venous return curve clockwise (not shown in Fig. 1.4)
  b. By decreasing the afterload (haemodilution and reduction in viscosity of the blood) and shifting the cardiac function curve towards the left (not shown in Fig. 1.4)

- In cases of a poorly contractile heart, the cardiac function curve is shifted downwards and towards the right. Even if the venous return curve is shifted towards left post fluid bolus, there is minimal or no change in CO. As can be seen in Fig. 1.4, despite shifting in the equilibrium point from point C to point D, there is no increase in cardiac output. Furthermore, as can be seen again in Fig. 1.4 there is a disproportionate increase in RAP with this fluid bolus (point C to point D in Fig. 1.4).
- An increase in RAP impedes the venous return (by decreasing the pressure gradient for VR). In addition, high RAP also produces back pressure changes and reduction in organ perfusion, by increasing renal, hepatic and intestinal venous pressure impairing in microcirculatory flow in those organs.
- Several experimental studies have reasonably substantiated these concepts of Guyton, as shown in Boxes 1.1 and 1.2.

**Box 1.1 Experiment by Cecconi et al.** [5]

- Cecconi and colleagues tested the Guytonian model of circulation in postoperative patients using Navigator™ technology. They tested the effects of fluid challenge on $P_{msa}$ (a $P_{ms}$ analogue) and venous return gradient (dVR = $P_{msa}$ – CVP). [CVP = Central Venous Pressure, a surrogate of RAP.]
- They found that in fluid responders (in whom fluid challenge increases cardiac output by >10%), fluid challenge was associated with a corresponding increase in dVR and minimal change in CVP. In contrast, dVR did not increase in non-responders despite a significant increase in $P_{ms}$, because of a disproportionate rise in CVP.
- Findings of Cecconi and colleagues further validate the Guytonian model.

**Box 1.2 Experiment by Mass et al.** [6]

- In postoperative cardiac surgery patients, Maas and colleagues reconstructed the venous return curve by constructing a regression line between pairs of cardiac output (as a surrogate of venous return) and central venous pressure (CVP as a surrogate of RAP), measured during inspiratory hold manoeuvre at different levels of plateau pressure. Their aim was to see the effects of intravascular volume status on $P_{ms}$.
- They measured the $P_{ms}$ at the intercept of venous return curve at *X*-axis (as discussed during a discussion on venous return curve).
- By constructing venous return curves, at baseline (in resting state), with head of the bed at 30 degrees (relative hypovolemia) and after infusion of 500 ml colloids, they could confirm that $P_{ms}$ decreases with hypovolemia and increases with hypervolemia, as expected from Guytonian model.

- **Effect of Vasoactive Drugs:** Vasopressors can both shift the venous return curve rightwards (by decreasing venous capacitance and increasing $P_{ms}$) and counter-clockwise (by increasing RVR) (not shown in Fig. 1.4). Overall effect of vasopressor on venous return (and cardiac output) depends on intravascular volume status.
  - In conditions with profound vasoplegia and relative increase in unstressed volume, vasopressor infusion can convert unstressed volume to stressed volume with a predominant rightward shift of the venous return curve [7].
- Inotropic infusion shifts the cardiac function curve to the left. With this changed cardiac function curve, an increase

in $P_{ms}$ (and venous return) will increase cardiac output further (point E to point F in Fig. 1.4).

## 1.8 Some Caveats

- Fluid bolus may not increase the cardiac output in every patient. As can be seen from the above discussion, in order to increase cardiac output, fluid bolus must increase the $P_{ms}$ with minimal change in right atrial pressure. At the same time, both right and left ventricles must work in the steep part of the cardiac function curve.
  - In clinical studies of patients with septic shock, only 50% of patients increase their cardiac output following fluid bolus [8].
- Increase in cardiac output and other hemodynamic benefits seen after rapid fluid bolus are very often only transient even in healthy volunteers.
  - Nunes and colleagues investigated the hemodynamic effects of 500 ml Crystalloid bolus over a period of 90 min in 20 critically ill patients [9]. In the overall patient population, after an initial increase post fluid bolus, the cardiac index (CI, defined as cardiac output per metre$^2$ body surface area) decreased to baseline value at 90 min.
  - Even in fluid responders (13 of 20 patients in whom CO increased to >15% from baseline post-fluid bolus), the initial increment in CI nearly disappeared at 90 min.
  - This lack of sustained benefit post fluid bolus can be explained by fluid extravasation to tissues and the latter is accentuated further in sick patients with endothelial dysfunction.
- Increase in Cardiac Output does not ensure improvement in oxygen delivery ($DO_2$) to the tissues, as $DO_2$ is determined also by haemoglobin level in blood and oxygen saturation of haemoglobin.

- Improvement in cardiac output and other macro-hemodynamic parameters do not ensure improved oxygen utilization at tissue level ($VO_2$) because of dysfunction at the level of microcirculation and mitochondria [10].
- Fluid bolus may fail to improve haemodynamics but it never fails to get accumulated in the body. Several studies have shown a strong association between cumulative positive fluid balance and adverse patient outcomes [11, 12].
- Finally, the publication of landmark "**FEAST**" Study performed in African children (discussed in Box 1.3) questions the benefit of fluid bolus itself and even raises concern about the safety of this strategy [13]. However, the results of this study need to be validated externally in resource-rich settings and amongst adult population.

**Box 1.3 "FEAST" Study** [13]

- **Research Question**: Is there any benefit of "Fluid Bolus" compared to "No Bolus" or whether there is any benefit of "Albumin Bolus" over "Saline Bolus" for early resuscitation in children from resource-poor settings.
- **Setting:** 11-Centres from Kenya, Tanzania and Uganda.
- **Patient:** 3141 Children (60 days to 12 years) with febrile illness complicated by impaired consciousness, respiratory distress or both and evidence of hypoperfusion (prolonged CRT >3 Second, lower limb temperature gradient, weak radial pulse or heart rate > 180/min).
- **Intervention:** Randomized in 1:1:1 ratio into one of the three following groups:
  - **Albumin Bolus:** Rapid bolus of 20–40 ml/Kg 5% Albumin within 1 hour followed by maintenance infusion of 2.5–4 ml/kg/hour maintenance fluid.

- **Saline Bolus:** Rapid bolus of 20–40 ml/Kg 5% 0.9% Saline within 1 hour followed by maintenance infusion of 2.5–4 ml/kg/hour maintenance fluid.
- **No Bolus:** Only maintenance fluid.

- **Outcome:**
  - The study was discontinued after the recruitment of 3141 (of proposed 3600 patients) in view of more harm observed in the bolus groups.
  - 48-hour mortality (Primary End-point) was significantly higher in both bolus groups compared to no bolus group (10.6% in Albumin-bolus, 10.5% in Saline-bolus and 7.3% in No-bolus groups).
  - Relative risk was not different between albumin bolus and saline bolus groups.
  - 4-week mortality remained higher in both bolus groups.
  - The results were consistent across centres and across subgroups.

## 1.9 Case Scenario (Continued)

- There are three possible hemodynamic effects of bolus Ringer's lactate on Mrs. RJ:
  - There may be an increase in stressed volume and $P_{ms}$ with minimal rise in RAP, increasing gradient to venous return, venous return itself and cardiac output. This in turn may improve organ perfusion.
  - Because of extreme vasoplegia, stressed volume and $P_{ms}$ may not increase. In the long run, this may harm Mrs. RJ by producing positive cumulative fluid balance.

– There may be some rise in $P_{ms}$ with a disproportionate increase in RAP and no change in venous return gradient. Rise in RAP may reduce the organ perfusion further as discussed earlier.

**Take-Home Messages**

- Rapid fluid bolus can improve haemodynamics in shock state by an increase in cardiac output, provided there is an increase in mean systemic pressure, minimal change in right atrial pressure and both ventricles are working in the steep portion of the cardiac function curve.
- Improvement in macro-hemodynamic does not ensure an increase in delivery of oxygen to tissues or utilization of oxygen in tissues.
- Potential harms associated with fluid bolus cannot be ignored and need to be considered before the prescription.

# References


1. Bayliss WM, Starling EH. Observations on venous pressures and their relationship to capillary pressures. J Physiol Lond. 1894;16:159–318.7.
2. Guyton AC, Lindsey AW, Abernathy B, Richardson T. Venous return at various right atrial pressures and the normal venous return curve. Am J Phys. 1957;189:609–15.
3. Patterson SW, Starling EH. On the mechanical factors which determine the output of the ventricles. J Physiol. 1914;48:357–79.
4. Guyton AC, Coleman TG, Granger HJ. Circulation: overall regulation. Annu Rev Physiol. 1972;34:13–46.
5. Cecconi M, Aya HD, Geisen M, Fletcher N, Grounds RM, Rhodes A. Changes in the mean systemic filling pressure during a fluid challenge in postsurgical intensive care patients. Intensive Care Med. 2013;39:1299–305.

6. Maas JJ, Geerts BF, van den Berg PC, Pinsky MR, Jansen JR. Assessment of venous return curve and mean systemic filling pressure in postoperative cardiac surgery patients. Crit Care Med. 2009;37:912–8.
7. Persichini R, Silva S, Teboul JL, Jozwiak M, Chemla D, Richard C, Monnet X. Effects of norepinephrine on mean systemic pressure and venous return in human septic shock. Crit Care Med. 2012;40:3146–53.
8. Marik PE, Cavallazzi R, Vasu T, Hirani A. Dynamic changes in arterial waveform derived variables and fluid responsiveness in mechanically ventilated patients: a systematic review of the literature. Crit Care Med. 2009;37:2642–7.
9. Nunes TS, Ladeira RT, Bafi AT, de Azevedo LCP, Machado FR, Freitas FGR. Duration of hemodynamic effects of crystalloids in patients with circulatory shock after initial resuscitation. Ann Intensive Care. 2014 Aug 1;4:25. https://doi.org/10.1186/s13613-014-0025-9.
10. Hernández G, Teboul JL. Is the macrocirculation really dissociated from the microcirculation in septic shock? Intensive Care Med. 2016;42:1621–4.
11. Boyd JH, Forbes J, Nakada TA, Walley KR, Russell JA. Fluid resuscitation in septic shock: a positive fluid balance and elevated central venous pressure are associated with increased mortality. Crit Care Med. 2011;39:259–65.
12. Silversides JA, Fitzgerald E, Manickavasagam US, Lapinsky SE, Nisenbaum R, Hemmings N, et al. Role of active deresuscitation after resuscitation (RADAR) investigators. Deresuscitation of patients with iatrogenic fluid overload is associated with reduced mortality in critical illness. Crit Care Med. 2018;46:1600–7.
13. Maitland K, Kiguli S, Opoka RO, Engoru C, Olupot-Olupot P, Akech SO, et al. Mortality after fluid bolus in African children with severe infection. N Engl J Med. 2011;364:2483–95.

# Chapter 2
# Compartmentalization Body Fluids. Regulation of Fluid Balance

## 2.1 Case Scenario

Mr. AL, a 43-year-old, otherwise healthy male, is having several loose bowel movements since morning. The stool is of large volume, watery and not associated with any blood or mucous. He does not have any fever or pain in abdomen and denies any history suggestive of possible food poisoning.

### *2.1.1 How Does Human Being Compensate for Loss of Body Fluid?*

Water constitutes a large proportion of our body weight. As we evolved from unicellular to a multicellular organism, the water content of our body is compartmentalized, with variable electrolyte and other solute concentrations in different compartments. This compartmentalization is required to maintain the metabolic needs of individual cells. For the same metabolic requirement, human beings (and other multicellular organisms) also need to maintain a tight balance between individual compartments **("Internal Balance"),** as well as with the environment surrounding our body (**"External Balance").** In this chapter, we shall discuss different body fluid compartments, their composition and how is the internal and external fluid balance maintained.



S. Ghosh, *Handbook of Intravenous Fluids*,
https://doi.org/10.1007/978-981-19-0500-1_2

## 2.2 Body Fluid Compartments

- Total water content of the human body is variable and depends on age, weight and gender. Water content of the body for an adult male and an adult female is approximately 60% and 50% of the bodyweight, respectively. In contrast, water constitutes up to 80% of the body weight in neonates. In other extreme of age, for an elderly male or an elderly female, it is about 50% and 45% of bodyweight, respectively.
- Approximately two/third of the total body water remains within the cell (or **Intracellular Fluid, ICF**).
- Remaining one/third water content of human body (or **Extracellular Fluid, ECF**) is again compartmentalized into three compartments—**Interstitial Fluid**, **Intravascular Fluid** and **Transcellular Fluid**.
  - Three/fourth of the extracellular fluid is in the interstitial compartment that is present in the tissues surrounding each and every cell—Interstitial Fluid.
  - Blood present in the intravascular compartment makes up around 5–6% of human body, out of which 55% is in liquid state (i.e. plasma).
  - Transcellular fluids are specialized fluids that surround different organs to maintain their integrity, for example pleural fluid, pericardial fluid, cerebrospinal fluid or fluids inside the joint spaces.

- Figure 2.1 depicts the approximate distribution of different fluid compartments in a 70-kg adult male.
- There are gross variations in the electrolyte composition of different body fluid compartments and are shown in Table 2.1.
- As can be seen in Table 2.1, extracellular fluid concentrations of Sodium and accompanying anion Chloride are significantly higher compared to intracellular fluid. As if all our cells are still floating in primitive seawater.

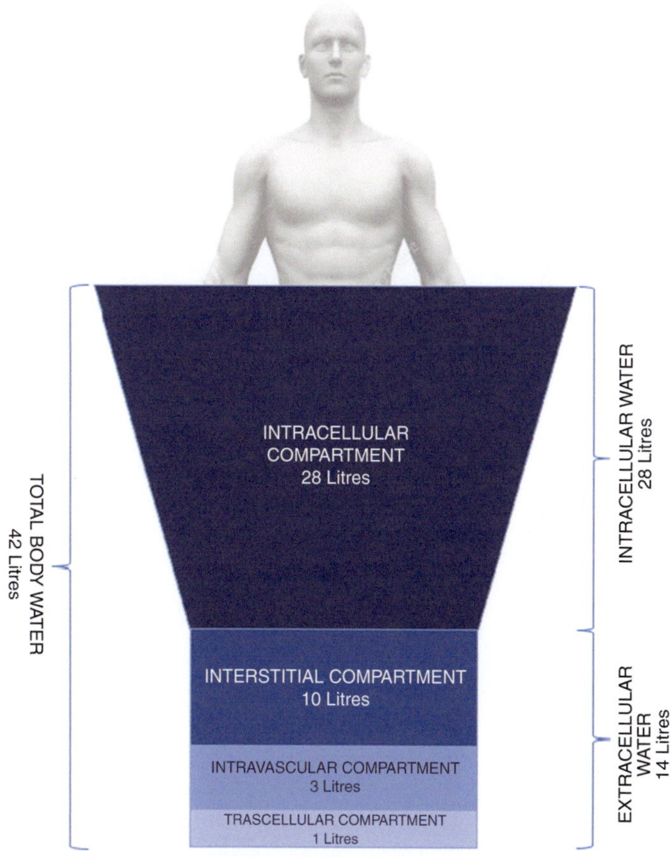


FIGURE 2.1 Approximate distribution of body water in an adult male weighing 70 kg

- Life started in the sea with unicellular organisms deriving their nutrition and oxygen from saline water. As we evolved from unicellular to a multicellular organism, cells still required to derive their nourishment from sodium rich fluids.
- With further evolution, higher organisms started carrying saline water within them (as can be seen in Fig. 2.2). Every cell in our body is still bathed by saline water

TABLE 2.1 Electrolyte composition of different fluid compartments

| | Intracellular fluid | Extracellular fluid | |
|---|---|---|---|
| | | Interstitial fluid | Plasma |
| Sodium (mEq/L) | 10 | 142 | 145 |
| Potassium (mEq/L) | 140 | 4 | 4 |
| Calcium (mEq/L) | <1 | 3 | 3 |
| Magnesium (mEq/L) | 50 | 2 | 2 |
| Chloride (mEq/L) | 4 | 110 | 105 |
| Bicarbonate (mEq/L) | 10 | 28 | 24 |
| Phosphorus (mEq/L) | 75 | 2 | 2 |
| Protein (gm/L) | **16** | **2** | **7** |

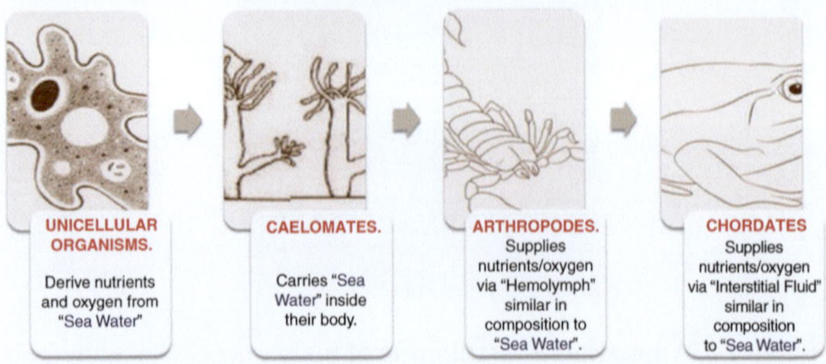


FIGURE 2.2 With evolution, we are only made to carry seawater along

(interstitial fluid), derives nutrition from the same and excretes the products of metabolism into it.

– In this environment, cells maintain their primeval capacity to keep sodium out of it and maintain their relatively high potassium content inside by an energy-dependent active $Na^+/K^+$-ATPase pump, present in the membranes of every cell.

- More evolved organisms (like human beings) have also developed a robust system to preserve the salinity of the extracellular fluid even in extremes of circumstances (discussed later in this chapter).

## 2.3 Essential Terminologies

- To understand subsequent paragraphs, we need to understand some essential terminologies, as discussed below.
- **Solvent:** A solvent is any substance into which another substance (or solute) is dissolved and forms a solution. A solution takes the same physical form (liquid, solid or gaseous) as the solvent. To form a solution, certain physical bond is developed between solute(s) and solvent.
- **Mixture:** A mixture is where substances are added to one another but they remain separate without any physical or chemical bond formed between them. All fluid compartments inside our body are quite complex containing both solutions (e.g. $Na^+$, $K^+$, $Cl^+$, urea, glucose, etc. dissolved in water) and mixtures (proteins, fats in water).
- **Osmole:** Osmole is a unit for measuring osmotic pressure (described later in the chapter) and defined as one-gram molecular weight of any substance in a solution. One osmole contains $6.022 \times 10^{23}$ ("**Avogadro Number**") particles of that particular substance. Milli-osmole is 1/1000th of an osmole.
- **Osmolarity:** Osmolarity is defined as the number of osmoles of a particular solute present per unit volume of a solution and is described as Osmoles/Litres. Solutes are present in human body fluids in much lower concentrations and are quantified as milliosmoles/Litre.
- **Osmolality:** Osmolality, on the contrary, is defined as the number of osmoles of a particular solute present per unit weight of a solvent and is described in body fluid as milliosmoles/kg of water.

  - Osmolarity and osmolality are often used interchangeably. But, since the volume of a solution is affected by temperature, it is preferable to use osmolality to describe the quantity of solute particles in body fluids.

- Osmolality of plasma can be calculated from the major solutes present in it and is described as calculated Osmolality.

$$\text{Calculated Plasma Osmolality} = 2 \times Na^{+} \text{ (in mosmol/Kg of water)} + \text{Plasma Glucose (in mg/dl)}/18 + \text{Blood Urea Nitrogen (in mg/dl)}/2.8$$

- Plasma osmolality can actually be measured by the freezing point depression method, when it is called measured osmolality.
- The difference between measured osmolality and calculated osmolality is usually <10 milliosmole/Kg of water. If it is more than that, one should suspect the presence of high concentration of other osmotically active substances (e.g. Toxic alcohols or Mannitol).
- Normal plasma osmolality is maintained within close range between 285 and 295 milliosmoles/kg of water.

- **Osmosis:** Osmosis is defined as a passive process (not dependent on energy) of movement of solvent from a solution of lower osmolality to the one with higher osmolality, when both these solutions are separated by a semipermeable membrane (a membrane which is selectively permeable to that particular solvent).
- **Tonicity:** Tonicity is defined as the relative concentration of osmotically active particles between two solutions separated by a semipermeable membrane.

  - Any particle that moves freely between two solutions through the membrane does not take part in osmosis and is not considered while defining tonicity. For example, glucose and urea move freely between intracellular and extracellular compartments and are not considered for the calculation of tonicity.
  - **Hypertonic:** Presence of a higher concentration of osmotically active solute in one side of the semipermeable membrane. If the extracellular fluid is hypertonic

(compared to intracellular fluid separated by semipermeable cell membrane), e.g. in the presence of hypernatremia or following mannitol infusion, water will move out of the intracellular compartment shrinking the cell.
  - **Hypotonic:** Presence of lower concentration of osmotically active solute in one side of the semipermeable membrane. Cells will swell in the presence of extracellular hypotonicity, e.g. in the presence of hyponatremia.
  - **Isotonic:** Concentration of osmotically active solutes in both sides of the membrane is equal.
  - To describe the tonicity of an intravenous fluid, it is compared with the tonicity of RBCs. Isotonic fluids are the ones which do not produce swelling or shrinkage of RBCs, when RBCs are suspended in them.

- **Diffusion:** Diffusion can be defined as the movement of a substance from a solution with higher concentration to the one with lower concentration through a permeable membrane.

## 2.4 Internal Balance

### *2.4.1 Movement Through Cell Membrane*

- Extracellular fluid compartment is separated from intracellular compartment by semipermeable cell membrane. Movement between these compartments takes place by the following means:
  - **Simple diffusion:** Cell membrane is permeable to certain solutes like glucose or urea. They can freely move through the membrane along the concentration gradient.
  - **Transmembrane channels:** Movement of electrolytes takes place through transmembrane channel. This is an energy-dependent process.

- **Osmosis:** Extracellular and intracellular fluids are isosmotic in steady state. Water can move from one compartment to another only if tonicity of one compartment changes.

- In physiological state, changes in tonicity can only be transiently related to movements of electrolytes through a transmembrane channel.
- But in pathological states, tonicity can change for a sustained period in different conditions. For example, the syndrome of inappropriate secretion of ant-diuretic hormone (SIADH) produces hyponatremia and hypotonicity of extracellular fluid compartment, resulting in the movement of water from extracellular to intracellular fluid along the osmotic gradient. Even in those situations, cells compensate slowly by reducing intracellular tonicity by removing proteins from the cells.
  - Change in extracellular tonicity can also be iatrogenic by infusion of hypotonic (5% Dextrose) or hypertonic (3% Saline or 20% Mannitol) fluid.

### *2.4.2 Movement Through Capillary Walls*

- Movement of solutes or water through capillary wall is mostly passive by either filtration or simple diffusion. Traditional view of the movement through capillary wall is dominated by "**Starling Concept**" described below.
  - Plasma is separated from the interstitial spaces by fenestrated capillary walls, which acts as a semipermeable membrane. Net movement of fluid from plasma to interstitial compartment depends on the balance between hydrostatic and oncotic pressure gradients within the capillary lumen and the interstitial fluid.
  - "**Starling Equation**" (stated below) mathematically expresses the balance between differing forces that determines the movement of fluid across capillary membranes:

$$J_v = L_p S[(P_c - P_i) - \sigma(\pi_c - \pi_i)]$$

- ($Jv$ = Transcapillary Flow, $L_p$ S = Permeability coefficient of the capillary surface, $\sigma$ = Reflection coefficient for protein permeability, $(P_c - P_i)$ = Capillary–interstitial hydrostatic pressure gradient, $(\pi_c - \pi_i)$ = Capillary–interstitial oncotic pressure gradient)
- **Starling Concept:** According to this concept, fluid is filtered out of capillaries to the interstitial spaces at the arteriolar end predominantly because of the higher hydrostatic pressure difference.
  - Hydrostatic pressure at the arteriolar end is approximately 32 mmHg. Whereas, hydrostatic pressure in the interstitial space is between −5 to 0 mmHg (with the exception of encapsulated organs where hydrostatic pressure of interstitial spaces is much higher).
  - At the venular end of capillaries, fluid is absorbed back to intravascular space because of the dominant colloid oncotic pressure gradient favouring movement towards the capillary lumen. Oncotic pressure in the capillaries is much higher (~25 mmHg) compared to interstitial spaces (~5 mmHg).
  - Starling concept is pictorially shown in Fig. 2.3.

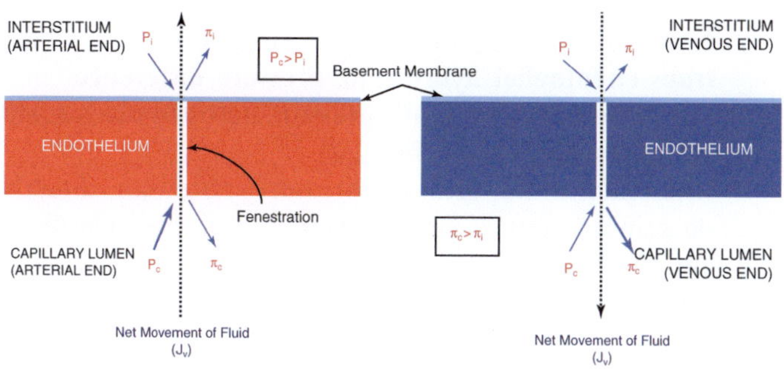


FIGURE 2.3 Cartoon illustrating Starling concept. *Jv* transcapillary flow, $P_c$ capillary hydrostatic pressure, $P_i$ interstitial hydrostatic pressure, $\pi_c$ capillary oncotic pressure, $\pi_i$ interstitial oncotic pressure

- However, with the discovery of glycocalyx, the concept of reabsorption of fluid at the venular end is put into question [1].

- **Endothelial Glycocalyx:** Endothelial Glycocalyx (EGL) is a mesh of membrane-bound glycoproteins and proteoglycans present at the luminal side of the entire vascular system. EGL layer separates RBCs and large proteins from the subendothelial space. The thickness and continuity of the glycocalyx layer are variable and depend on the type of vessels.
  - EGL is thinner in the microcirculation and much thicker in larger vessels.
  - Over fenestrated areas of capillaries, EGL layers are comparatively thinner. For the same reason, EGL layer is more discontinuous in tissues with highly fenestrated capillaries (e.g. hepatic sinusoids) compared to tissues like nervous systems or muscles.
  - Fluids in the sub-glycocalyx compartment are almost devoid of protein with very low oncotic pressure.

- **Revised Starling Concept:** With the discovery of glycocalyx layer and the understanding of sub-glycocalyx fluid compartment participating in the movement of fluid in and out of capillary lumen, original Starling concept needed revision.
  - New concept proposes revised Starling forces as "**the trans-endothelial hydrostatic pressure difference**" and "**the difference in osmotic pressure between plasma and sub-glycocalyx fluid**" (Fig. 2.4).
  - Interstitial fluid osmotic pressure does not directly determine net fluid movement across capillary endothelium.
  - Furthermore, with almost negligible oncotic pressure in the sub-glycocalyx fluid compartment, net lumen-ward movement of fluid at the venular end of capillaries is much lower compared to that postulated by original Starling concept.

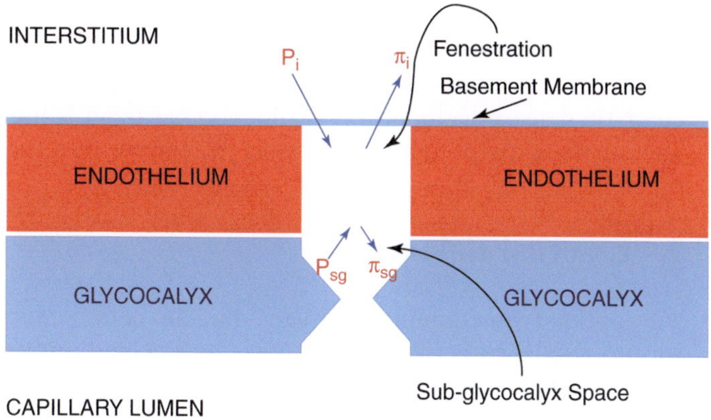


FIGURE 2.4 Cartoon illustrating endothelial glycocalyx and sub-glycocalyx space. $P_i$ interstitial hydrostatic pressure, $\pi_i$ interstitial oncotic pressure, $P_{sg}$ hydrostatic pressure within sub-glycocalyx space, $\pi sg$ osmotic pressure within sub-glycocalyx space

- **Inflammatory States:** Glycocalyx layer is damaged in inflammatory states like sepsis, burn, pancreatitis, diabetes mellitus—significantly increasing the movement of fluid out of capillary lumen.
  - Increasing capillary osmotic pressure (e.g. by infusion of colloids like albumin) can only dehydrate the sub-glycocalyx space by increasing the osmotic pressure gradient between intravascular compartment and sub-glycocalyx compartment. But the net movement of fluid from the interstitium towards capillary lumen will be only minimal (if at all).
  - Proteins (especially albumin) are also filtered out of capillary lumen through large fenestrations (for example in hepatic sinusoids) or through endothelial channels. This movement of proteins out of capillary lumen is increased in inflammatory states.
- **Lymphatics:** Fluid (also albumin and other proteins) is moved back to intravascular space through lymphatic channels. This flow of fluid and albumin from interstitial

space to the intravascular compartment can be increased in inflammatory state; but only up to a certain limit. Beyond that limit any further movement of fluid from interstitial space to the intravascular compartment is limited significantly; potentially increasing interstitial oedema.

## 2.5 External Balance

- For optimal functioning of organs, human beings must ensure a balance between total intake and overall output of fluids and electrolytes, so that volumes of different body compartments are maintained.
- In health, body fluids are lost via urine, through gastrointestinal tract (faeces) or through insensible loss from sweat and respiration. Insensible loss depends on ambient temperature and body's metabolic activities. Lost volume is replaced by oral intake (stimulated by thirst mechanism) or from water generated from metabolic activities.
- Table 2.2 gives an approximate estimate of the output and intake of a 70-kg healthy male.
- Electrolytes are constantly being lost through different ways and must be replaced through adequate intake. Table 2.3 provides an estimate of electrolytes lost from the body on a daily basis (and requirement).

TABLE 2.2 Daily water balance in health

| **Daily output** | | **Daily intake** | |
|---|---|---|---|
| Urine | 1500 ml | Drinking | 1500 ml |
| Gastrointestinal | 200 ml | Solid food | 750 ml |
| Skin (sweat) | 400 ml | From metabolism | 250 ml |
| Respiratory | 400 ml | | |
| Total | 2500 ml | Total | 2500 ml |

TABLE 2.3 Daily loss of electrolytes in health

| Electrolytes | Daily loss (and requirements) |
|---|---|
| Sodium | 1–1.5 mmol/kg body weight |
| Potassium | 1–1.5 mmol/kg body weight |
| Magnesium | 0.1–0.2 mmol/kg body weight |
| Calcium | 0.1–0.2 mmol/kg body weight |
| Chloride | 0.07–0.22 mmol/kg body weight |
| Phosphate | 20–40 mmol/kg body weight |

## 2.6 Hypovolemia and Body's Response

- With a scarce source of water (and sodium) in the atmosphere outside the seawater, it was necessary for human beings to develop a vast defence system to conserve water (and sodium) for maintaining extracellular fluid volume. In the following paragraphs, we shall discuss these defence mechanisms in brief.
- **Thirst Mechanism:** Hypovolemia activates the low-pressure mechanoreceptors present in atria and pulmonary vessels, which in turn send a signal to thirst centres located in the hypothalamus.
  - Thirst centre is also activated by any increase in plasma osmolality (an inevitable consequence of volume loss). These highly sensitive osmoreceptors are present in the organum vasculosum of the lamina terminalis (OVLT) and sub-fornical organ within the hypothalamus.
  - Stimulation of thirst mechanism increases oral intake (provided there is ready access to the same).
- **Sympathetic System:** Hypovolemia produces a reduction in venous return, fall in cardiac output and a drop in arterial blood pressure. Fall in blood pressure stimulates baroreceptors present in carotid sinuses and aortic arch and produces sympathetic stimulation.

  - Sympathetic stimulation also results from the activation of chemoreceptors that senses systemic acidosis resulting from a fall in tissue blood flow.
  - Increased sympathetic activity stimulates the adrenal medulla to release noradrenaline in the blood. Noradrenaline causes constriction of both afferent and efferent arterioles reducing glomerular filtration rate (GFR). As a consequence, excretion of both water and $Na^+$ is reduced.

- **Anti-diuretic Hormone (ADH):** ADH, also known as vasopressin, is synthesized in the supraoptic and paraventricular nuclei of the hypothalamus and is transported to the posterior pituitary via the neurohypophysial capillaries, where it is stored.
  - In cases of hypovolemia and more importantly, with an increase in plasma osmolality, hypothalamus sends a signal to the posterior pituitary to release the hormone.
  - ADH facilitates the reabsorption of water from the collecting ducts of the nephrons.
  - ADH binds to the V2 receptors at the luminal side of the collecting ducts, which in turn results in the insertion of aquaporin 2 in the luminal walls. Insertion of aquaporin 2 makes the otherwise impermeable collecting ducts to reabsorb water along the osmotic gradient present in renal medulla.
  - In addition, ADH also produces arterial vasoconstriction via V2 receptors and plays an important role in maintaining systemic blood pressure in the presence of profound hypovolemia.

- **Renin–Angiotensin System (RAS):** Renin is a hormone released from the juxtaglomerular apparatus in response to any fall in $Na^+$ content of the tubular filtrate or in the presence of low afferent arteriolar pressure or from stimulation of sympathetic nervous system.

- Renin, in turn, cleaves angiotensinogen (a plasma protein synthesized in the liver) into angiotensin I.
- Angiotensin I is converted to angiotensin II by angiotensin-converting enzyme present predominantly in the capillaries of the lungs, but also in the endothelium of other vessels and renal tubular epithelium.
- Angiotensin II reduces the GFR by constriction of afferent (and also efferent) arterioles and increases $Na^+$ reabsorption from the proximal convoluted tubules (PCT) of the nephrons.
- Angiotensin II also triggers the release of aldosterone from the zona glomerulosa of the adrenal cortex. Aldosterone, in turn, acts on distal convoluted tubules (DCT) and collecting ducts of nephrons, promoting reabsorption of $Na^+$ (in exchange of $K^+$ and $H^+$) and water.
- Some minor roles of angiotensin II are triggering the release of ADH from posterior pituitary and promoting secretion of noradrenaline from sympathetic nerve endings.

• Figure 2.5 summarizes the body's response to hypovolemia.

## 2.7 Hypervolemia and Body's Response

• Compared to hypovolemia body's response to hypervolemia is much less robust.
• In addition to the reduced release of three hypovolemia hormones described above, **Atrial Natriuretic Peptide** (ANP) and **Brain-type Natriuretic Peptide** (BNP) are released predominantly from atria and ventricles, respectively, as they are stretched as a result of hypervolemia.
• ANP and BNP have number of effects albeit weak resulting in increased excretion of sodium and water.

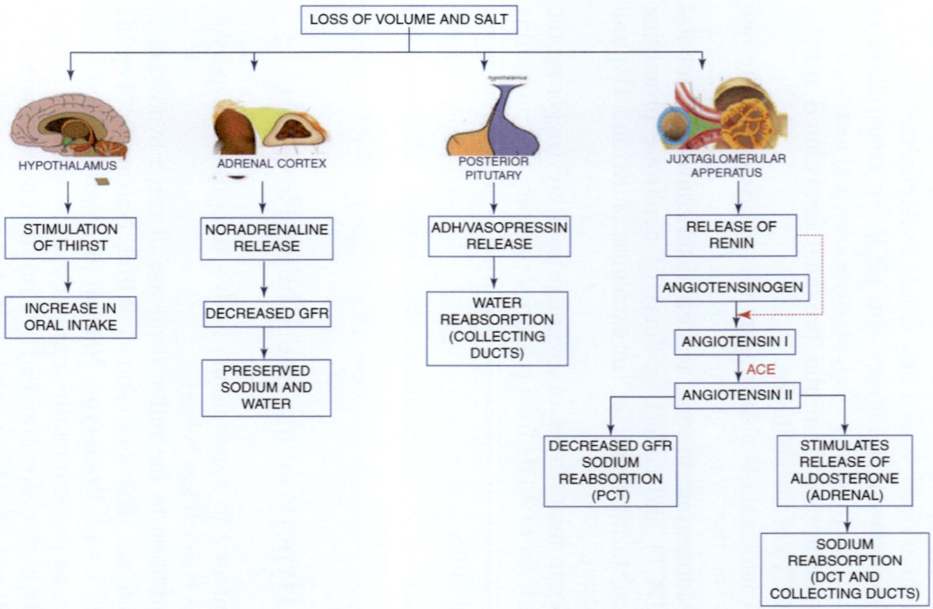


Figure 2.5 Schematic diagram showing response to hypovolemia. *GFR* glomerular filtration rate, *ADH* anti-diuretic hormone, *ACE* angiotensin-converting enzyme

- Increase in GFR and Na+ excretion by afferent arteriolar dilatation and efferent arteriolar constriction, thus increasing glomerular filtration pressure.
- They also increase the available surface area for glomerular filtration by relaxation of mesangial cells.
- They inhibit Na+ reabsorption from DCT.
- In addition, they also inhibit the secretion of renin and aldosterone.

## 2.8 Case Scenario (Continued)

- Hypovolemia in Mr. AL is due to diarrhoeal loss of fluid. This will initially be compensated by the physiological mechanism described above including an increase in oral fluid intake because of activation of thirst mechanism and secretion of three "hypovolemia hormones."
- However, beyond a certain limit, these physiological responses may not be able to compensate further, requiring medical intervention including intravenous fluid administration.
- In addition, appropriate treatment of the etiological factor for diarrhoea will be necessary to contain further fluid loss.

**Take-Home Messages**

- In this chapter, we have learned that human body consists mostly of water that itself is compartmentalized.
- We have also learned that a balance is maintained between different fluid compartments that are determined by different Starling forces.
- A fine balance is maintained with the surrounding environment, so that overall fluid volume remains constant inside the body. Robust mechanisms are in place to maintain that balance.

- Key point to understand is that salt and water preserving mechanisms are much stronger compared to salt and water excretory mechanisms. Unfortunately, the environment within the hospital is "salt rich" with a potential to produce iatrogenic "salt water drowning" by infusing too much sodium-containing intravenous fluid [2, 3].

## References

1. Woodcock TE, Woodcock TM. Revised Starling equation and the glycocalyx model of transvascular fluid exchange: an improved paradigm for prescribing intravenous fluid therapy. Br J Anaesth. 2012;108:384–94.
2. Van Regenmortel N, Moers L, Langer T, Roelant E, De Weerdt T, Caironi P, et al. Fluid-induced harm in the hospital: look beyond volume and start considering sodium. From physiology towards recommendations for daily practice in hospitalized adults. Ann Intensive Care. 2021;11:79.
3. Marik PE. Iatrogenic salt water drowning and the hazards of a high central venous pressure. Ann Intensive Care. 2014;4:21.

# Chapter 3
# Heart–Lung Interaction

## 3.1 Case Scenario

Mr. RR, a 67-year-old hypertensive gentleman with a past history of heavy smoking (stopped 2 years back for wheezy cough) was admitted for planned laparoscopic cholecystectomy. Two years ago, he underwent percutaneous transluminal coronary angioplasty (PTCA) with stent to left anterior descending coronary artery for chronic stable angina. During pre-operative evaluation, he had a normal size left ventricular cavity with no regional wall motion abnormality and LV ejection fraction of 55% on transthoracic echocardiography. Dobutamine Stress Echo was negative for inducible ischemia. Surgery was performed under general anaesthesia with an uneventful intra-operative course. Postoperatively he was extubated by the anaesthesia team following standard protocol. However, within a few minutes of extubation, he became acutely breathless with a regular heart rate of 128/min, blood pressure of 186/94 mmHg, respiratory rate of 28/min and pulse oximetry reading of 88% on 8 litres of oxygen by mask. He was immediately re-intubated and was shifted to ICU for further management. Chest X-ray done in the ICU showed bilateral infiltrate, centrally located around the hila, suggestive of acute pulmonary oedema.



S. Ghosh, *Handbook of Intravenous Fluids*,
https://doi.org/10.1007/978-981-19-0500-1_3

### *3.1.1 How Does Two Intra-thoracic Organs Heart and Lung, Interact with Each Other?*

Phasic changes of intrathoracic pressure during both spontaneous and positive pressure breathing effects stroke volume (SV), heart rate (HR), cardiac output (CO) and blood pressure (BP). Intrathoracic pressure changes impact the venous return or right ventricular preload, left ventricular preload, ventricular (both right and left) afterload with minimal or no effect on ventricular contractility. These effects can be transient during spontaneous breathing or more sustained during positive pressure breathing. In this chapter, we shall discuss the effects of respiratory phases on cardiac function, also known as heart–lung interaction and their implications in clinical practice.

## 3.2 Inspiration and Venous Return

- So far, we have learned that over any time frame longer than a few heartbeats cardiac output must be equal to venous return, i.e. whatever comes into the heart must be pumped out. We also have learned that venous return is directly proportional to the gradient between mean systemic filling pressure ($P_{ms}$, or the upstream pressure of venous return gradient) and right atrial pressure (RAP, or the downstream pressure of venous return gradient) and inversely proportional to the resistance to venous return (RVR). Venous return also depends on certain critical pressure ($P_{crit}$, or the intramural RAP below which transmural pressure of the great veins at the thoracic inlet becomes more negative than atmospheric pressure leading to their collapse, preventing further increase in venous return).
- Increase in intrathoracic pressure during positive pressure breathing, especially with high positive end-expiratory

pressure (PEEP, both intrinsic or extrinsic) produces the following changes to the determinants of venous return:

- Intramural RAP is increased impeding the venous return.
- Compensatory increase in $P_{ms}$ because of an enhancement of venous tone mediated by increased sympatho-adrenergic activity. Additionally, the mechanical effect of positive intrathoracic pressure produces downward movement of diaphragm, increasing intra-abdominal pressure and transfer of unstressed splanchnic blood to stressed volume. This increase in $P_{ms}$ at least partially counterbalances the effects of raised RAP on venous return gradient.
- RVR is increased.
- $P_{crit}$ is changed with PEEP because of the distorted geometry of venae cavae at the thoracic inlet, leading to earlier flattening of venous return curve.

• ***Overall, positive pressure breathing decreases venous return, especially in the inspiratory phase.*** This effect is more evident in the hypovolemic state, as hypovolemia can blunt the compensatory rise in $P_{ms}$.
• Opposite effect is expected to be seen in spontaneous inspiration.

## 3.3 Inspiration and Ventricular Afterload

• Ventricular afterload is defined as the force opposing ventricular ejection, represented by the transmural pressure within either aortic root (for left ventricle, LV) or pulmonary trunk (for right ventricle, RV), during ventricular systole. Transmural pressure is the difference between pressure inside the vessel or intramural pressure minus pressure outside of it (in this case pleural pressure).

### *3.3.1 LV Afterload During Spontaneous Breathing*

- Fall in intrathoracic pressure during spontaneous inspiration leads to a fall in both aortic root pressure and pleural pressure. But, compared to pleural pressure, fall in aortic root pressure is lower because of its connection with the extra-thoracic artery (abdominal aorta).
- This relative decrease in pleural pressure (pleural pressure more negative than aortic root pressure) compared to aortic root pressure results in an increase in transmural pressure at the aortic root during spontaneous inspiration.
- ***Net result increased left ventricular afterload during spontaneous inspiration.***
- Opposite effect is seen during spontaneous expiration (but with lesser intensity).

### *3.3.2 LV Afterload During Positive Pressure Breathing*

- Increase in intrathoracic pressure during positive pressure inspiration results in an increase in both aortic root pressure and pleural pressure. But increase in aortic root pressure is comparatively lesser than the increase in pleural pressure (following the same principle described in the previous section).
- This relative increase in pleural pressure compared to the aortic root pressure results in a fall in transmural pressure during positive pressure inspiration.
- ***Net result decreased left ventricular afterload during positive pressure inspiration.***
- During expiration, these changes are reversed.

### 3.3.3 *RV Afterload During Respiration*

- Increase in alveolar pressure during both spontaneous and positive pressure inspiration results in an increase in West Zone 1 and 2 conditions, as opposed to Zone 3 conditions.
- Zones 1 or 2 condition exists, whenever alveolar pressure ($P_A$) exceeds the intraluminal pressure of alveolar capillaries, either in the venous side ($P_v$) and/or in the arterial side ($P_a$) (Zone 1 = $P_A > P_a > P_v$. Zone 2 = $P_a > P_A > P_v$), resulting in vessel compression. By contrast, in Zone 3 condition intraluminal capillary pressure exceeds alveolar pressure (Zone 3 = $P_a > P_v > P_A$).
- ***Increase in Zone 1 and 2 conditions during inspiration lead to an increase in pulmonary artery pressure and thus right ventricular afterload during both spontaneous and positive pressure inspiration.***

## 3.4 Inspiration and Ventricular Interdependence

- Right and left ventricles share a common septum and circumferential fibres. Moreover, expansion of both ventricles is restrained by a common pericardium. For these reasons, the shape and stiffness of one ventricle is significantly affected by the diastolic filling of the other ventricle. This phenomenon is known as ventricular parallel interdependence.
- On the other hand, diastolic filling of left ventricle is dependent on the right ventricular output. This propagation of changes in right ventricular output on left ventricular output because of the series arrangement of both ventricles is known as ventricular series interdependence.

### 3.4.1 Ventricular Parallel Interdependence

- Increase in venous return and RV filling during spontaneous inspiration leads to a leftward shift of the interventricular septum and a stiffer LV. ***This parallel effect of ventricular diastolic interdependence leads to a decrease in LV preload and a fall in LV Stroke Volume, Pulse Pressure and Systolic Pressure during spontaneous inspiration.***
- Opposite effect is seen in positive pressure breathing. With a fall in venous return, RV size decreases resulting in a shift of septum towards right, a decrease in LV wall stiffness and an increase in LV preload. This LV preload effect is further augmented by an increase in pulmonary venous drainage produced by the squeezing effect of raised intrathoracic pressure during positive pressure inspiration. ***This increase in LV preload during positive pressure inspiration leads to an increase in LV Stroke Volume, Pulse Pressure and Systolic Pressure.***

### 3.4.2 Ventricular Series Interdependence

- Increase in right ventricular afterload during spontaneous inspiration exaggerates the fall in left ventricular preload (due to parallel effect).
- During positive pressure inspiration, following an initial increase in LV preload (due to parallel ventricular interdependence), preload decreases after 3–4 heartbeats, resulting from a fall in RV Stroke Volume during positive pressure breathing.
- ***This ventricular series interdependence ultimately leads to a decrease in LV Stroke Volume, Pulse Pressure and Systolic Pressure, during the later part of inspiration and during expiration.***
- Fall in LV stroke volume and arterial pressure during later part of positive pressure inspiration and expiratory phase is more pronounced in patients with hypovolemia.

## 3.5 Heart–Lung Interaction: During Spontaneous Respiration

- Overall effect of spontaneous inspiration on right and left sides of the heart is schematically presented in Fig. 3.1.
- **Pulsus Paradoxus:** During quiet respiration in a healthy individual, inspiratory fall in systolic blood pressure (SBP) is usually less than 10 mmHg. However, in certain clinical conditions like acute severe asthma and cardiac tamponade, an abnormally large fall (by >10 mmHg) in SBP may be observed. This later phenomenon is termed "**Pulsus Paradoxus**".
  - Mechanisms of pulsus paradoxus, however, may differ in different conditions.
  - Primary mechanism of pulsus paradoxus in cardiac tamponade is a large increase in parallel diastolic ventricular interdependence effect within the pressurized pericardium, resulting in an excessive decrease in LV preload. In fact, pulsus paradoxus may be minimal or absent, when cardiac tamponade is associated with an underlying atrial/ventricular septal defect or a dilated dysfunctional left ventricle.

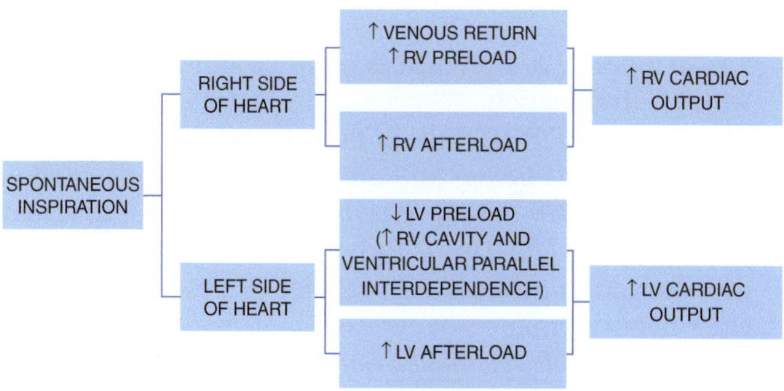


FIGURE 3.1 Effect of spontaneous inspiration on cardiac output during quiet breathing

– The predominant mechanism of pulsus paradoxus in acute severe asthma is a decrease in LV preload as a result of a fall in RV Stroke Volume. Fall in RV Stroke Volume, in turn, is because of a disproportionate increase in RV afterload resulting from extreme hyperinflation.

- In young healthy individuals, heart rate varies in phases of respiration. During inspiratory phase, heart rate increases due to reflex inhibition of vagal tone. In contrast, initiation of expiratory phase restores the vagal tone resulting in a decrease in heart rate. This respirophasic variation in heart rate is known as "**Sinus Arrhythmia**".

## 3.6 Heart–Lung Interaction: During Positive Pressure Breathing

- Overall effects of positive pressure breathing on both sides of the heart are schematically depicted in Fig. 3.2.
- As can be seen in Fig. 3.2, LV output or stroke volume (SV) increases in the early stage of positive pressure inspiration, because of a fall in LV afterload and an increase in LV preload (pulmonary venous blood getting squeezed out and parallel ventricular interdependence). *This increase in LV SV during positive pressure inspiration and resulting increase in pulse pressure (PP) and SBP is termed "Δ Up Effect"*. Δ Up effect is more prominent in patients with LV dysfunction.
- LV SV (and PP/SBP) falls in the later stage of inspiration (after 3–4 heart beats) and during expiration. *This fall in LV SV/PP/SBP during late inspiratory and expiratory phase is termed "Δ Down Effect"*. Δ Down effect is more pronounced in patients with relative or absolute intravascular hypovolemia.
- *In a mechanically ventilated patient with evidence of tissue hypoperfusion, demonstration of a significant increase in Δ Down effect may suggest possible benefit of volume loading on cardiac output (so-called "fluid responsiveness").*

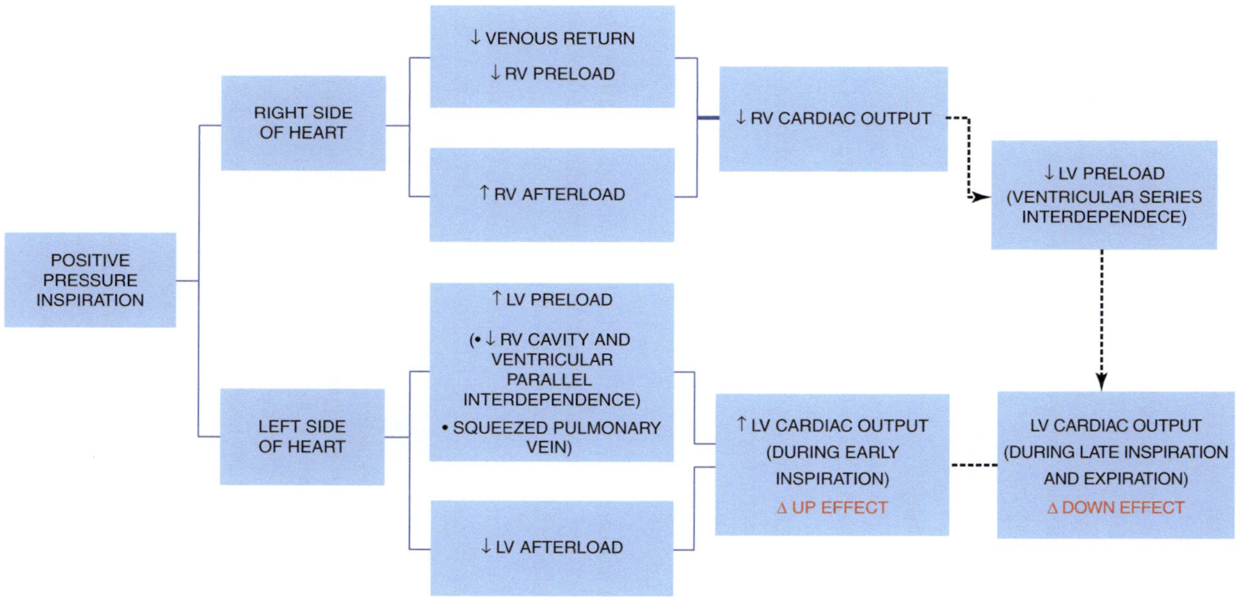


FIGURE 3.2 Effect of positive pressure breathing on cardiac output

## 3.7 Weaning Induced Pulmonary Oedema

- In 1988, Lemaire and colleagues described an interesting phenomenon while monitoring the haemodynamic status of 15 patients with COAD with underlying cardiovascular dysfunction on weaning trial with T-piece, using pulmonary artery catheter [1].
  - They observed a large increase in HR, arterial BP and cardiac index (CI) within 10 min of spontaneous breathing.
  - More importantly, the transmural Pulmonary Artery Occlusion Pressure (PAOP, a surrogate of LV filling pressure) increased from a mean value of 8 mmHg to 25 mmHg mandating the re-initiation of positive pressure ventilation.
  - These patients were treated with diuretics for 10 days and 9 of them could be successfully weaned off from ventilator.
- **Mechanism:** An increase in the work of breathing and associated anxiety activates the sympathetic response with an expected increase in HR and BP.
  - This increase in HR (with a decrease in diastolic cardiac perfusion time) and BP along with a decrease in arterial partial pressure of oxygen (PaO2) can precipitate myocardial ischemia (more likely in patients with underlying coronary artery disease).
  - Myocardial ischemia produces diastolic cardiac dysfunction and LV end diastolic pressure (LVEDP).
  - LVEDP is also increased during T-piece weaning trial because of an increase in both increase in LV preload (series interdependence) and LV afterload. Later effects are more pronounced again in patients with compromised LV function.
  - Increase in LVEDP during a spontaneous breathing trial on T-piece, especially in a patient with compromised LV function, can precipitate pulmonary oedema.

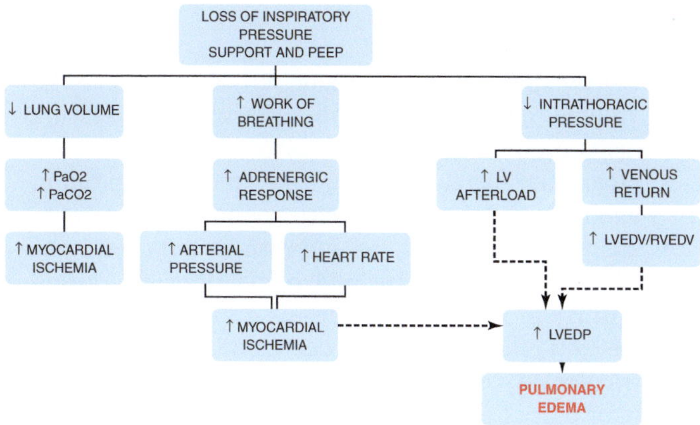


FIGURE 3.3 Effect of spontaneous breathing trial (T-Piece Trial) on cardiac function

- Overall effect of spontaneous breathing trial on cardiac function is schematically shown in Fig. 3.3.

## 3.8 Case Scenario (Continued)

- Mr. RR had weaning-induced pulmonary oedema. He should be worked up for perioperative myocardial ischemia.
- Management should include LV preload reduction with pulmonary venodilator (like nitroglycerin and furosemide) and diuretics, reduction of LV afterload with judicious use of vasodilator. Re-instituting positive pressure breathing will certainly help him and maybe life-saving too.
- With improvement in pulmonary oedema and optimization of overall condition, he may be weaned off or extubated early on non-invasive ventilatory support.

**Take-Home Messages**

- During spontaneous breathing, left ventricular stroke volume and arterial blood pressure fall during inspiration.
- Heart rate increases during spontaneous inspiration and falls during spontaneous expiration.
- ΔUp effect produces an increase in both left ventricular stroke volume and blood pressure, during positive pressure inspiration.
- ΔDown effect produces a decrease in both left ventricular stroke volume and blood pressure, during the later part of positive pressure inspiration and during expiratory phase.
- During T-piece weaning trial, especially in patients with underlying coronary artery disease, higher risk of myocardial ischemia, increased afterload and an increase in left ventricular end-diastolic volume, increases left ventricular end-diastolic pressure. This rise in LVEDP can lead to pulmonary oedema and weaning failure.

## Reference

1. Lemaire F, Teboul JL, Cinotti L, Giotto G, Abrouk F, Steg G, et al. Acute left ventricular dysfunction during unsuccessful weaning from mechanical ventilation. Anesthesiology. 1988;69:171–9.

# Chapter 4
# Acid–Base Physiology

## 4.1 Case Scenario

Mr. MJ, a 46-year-old male with a past history of alcoholic liver disease was admitted to the Intensive Care Unit with hypotension following variceal bleeding. On examination, he had evidence of circulatory shock. Blood gases done on admission showed: pH—7.40, $PaCO_2$—39 mmHg, $HCO_3$—24 mEq/L, BE—0. Laboratory reports revealed: Na—125 mEq/L, K—5.2 mEq/L, Cl—98 mEq/L, Albumin—13 g/L, Ca—3.2 mEq/L and Pi—1.5 mg/dl.

### *4.1.1 How to Elucidate Disturbances in Acid Base Balance (if Any) From the Given Clinical and Biochemical Information?*

Understanding acid–base physiology is fundamental to understanding the pathophysiology of a large number of clinical problems, especially so in the acute care setting. Analysis of blood gases (in conjunction with serum electrolytes) helps in decision-making regarding appropriate treatment and follow-up. Essentially acid–base disorders are classified into two broad categories—respiratory (when the



S. Ghosh, *Handbook of Intravenous Fluids*,
https://doi.org/10.1007/978-981-19-0500-1_4

primary abnormality involves respiration and partial pressure of carbon dioxide [$PaCO_2$] in plasma) and metabolic (when the primary abnormality is non-respiratory). There are three major approaches to acid–base interpretation—"**Traditional Approach**" (or so-called "**Physiological Approach**"), "**Stewart's Physicochemical Approach**" and "**Siggaard-Anderson's Base Excess Approach**". All three approaches more or less agree in their interpretation of respiratory disorder and differ only in their method of interpreting metabolic problems. In this chapter, we shall discuss the two most common approaches to acid–base abnormalities used in critical care settings—Traditional approach and Stewart's physicochemical approach.

## 4.2 Traditional Approach

- Despite its limitations, this approach remains the most popular way of interpreting acid–base disorders. It is based on the Henderson–Hasselbalch equation, which states that:

$$pH = pK + \log 10\left(\left[HCO_3 \cdot\right] \div \left[0.03 \times \left(PaCO_2\right)\right]\right) \quad (4.1)$$

(where, pH = Negative logarithm of [$H^+$] concentration. pK = Acid dissociation constant. [$HCO_3^-$] = Bicarbonate ion concentration in plasma in millimoles/litre. $PaCO_2$ = Partial pressure of $CO_2$ in mmHg)

- More simplistically, according to the traditional approach, [$H^+$] concentration is proportional to the ratio [$PaCO_2$]/[$HCO_3^-$]. An acid–base disorder is called "respiratory" when changes in [$H^+$] concentration is primarily because of changes in [$PaCO_2$] and "metabolic" when changes in [$H^+$] ion concertation is attributed to variation in [$HCO_3^-$].
- [$H^+$] concentration (and pH) is tightly regulated within the physiological range as virtually all human enzymes and membranes work best in this range. With any deviation in pH, the body tries to adapt and compensate, in an attempt

to maintain the pH. Compensatory changes in $PaCO_2$ and [$HCO_3^-$] in response to primary metabolic and respiratory disorder follows a pattern and can be predicted using empirical formulae. But remember compensatory responses can never normalize the pH, the only exception being chronic respiratory alkalosis.

  - With a primary metabolic problem, body compensates by altering respiratory drive. This respiratory compensation is quick and is activated within minutes.
  - In cases of primary respiratory disorders, kidneys adapt and change [$HCO_3^-$] concentration. This metabolic compensation (primarily by kidneys) is relatively slow, taking up to 5 days for complete adaptation.

- In subsequent paragraphs, we will discuss a 7-Step approach to acid–base disorders utilizing traditional approach.

**STEP 1: Starting point—History and physical examination**

- Clinical history and physical examination provide clue to underlying acid–base abnormalities. Some of the important clinical clues may be derived from:
- Underlying disease conditions: DM, Chronic pulmonary, renal or hepatic
- Presenting features: Circulatory shock, vomiting, diarrhoea
- Medication history: Diuretic, Metformin, Anti-Retroviral Drugs
- Ingestion of drugs or toxins

**STEP 2: Observe the pH, $PaCO_2$ and $HCO_3$**

- The purpose of this step is to look for any acid–base abnormality and to recognize a primary disorder (if any). Remember this so-called primary disorder is solely for the purpose of calculating compensatory response and not to give any undue importance to one disorder over another.
- For the analysis of acid–base abnormality using physiological approach we shall take normal values of pH as 7.40 ± 2, [$HCO_3^-$] as 24 ± 2 mmol/L and $PaCO_2$ as 40 ± 2 mmHg.
- Figure 4.1 describes a schema to identify any primary disorder from the given blood gas:

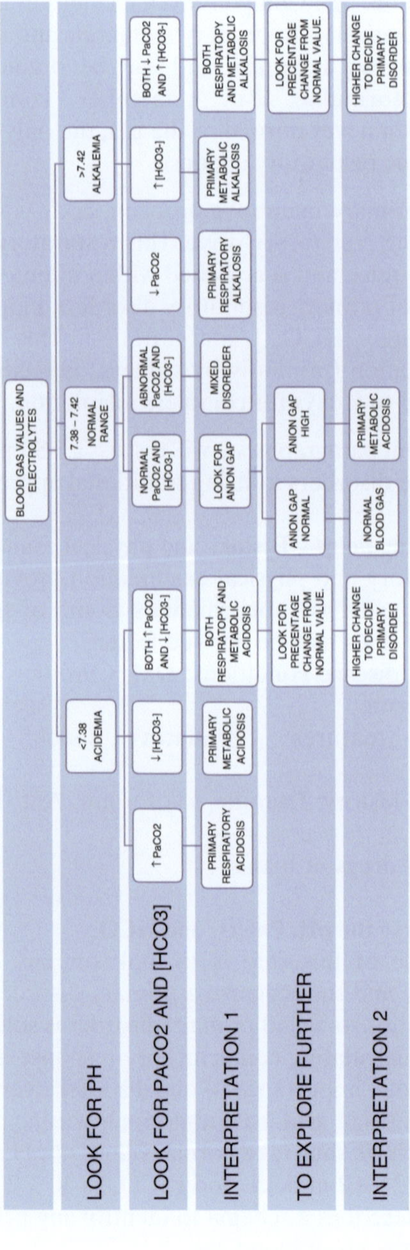


FIGURE 4.1 Look for primary disorder (traditional approach)

**STEP 3: Look for compensatory response**

- Compensatory responses (or expected change in $PaCO_2$ for any deviation of $[HCO_3-]$ from normal value and vice versa) are calculated based on empirical formulae. The whole purpose of this step is to identify a second disorder (if any).
- **Metabolic Acidosis**: If the primary disorder is metabolic acidosis, expected compensatory response is a fall in $PaCO_2$. Expected $PaCO_2$ in case of primary metabolic acidosis can be calculated from the following formula, also known as Winter's formula:

$$\text{Expected PaCO}_2 = \left(1.5 \times \left[\text{HCO}_3\right] + 8\right) \pm 2\,\text{mm Hg}\left(\text{Winter's Formula}\right) \quad (4.2)$$

  - If, measured $PaCO_2$ > Expected $PaCO_2$ = Additional Respiratory Acidosis.
  - If, measured $PaCO_2$ < Expected $PaCO_2$ = Additional Respiratory Alkalosis.

- **Metabolic Alkalosis:** If the primary disorder is metabolic alkalosis, expected response is an increase in $PaCO_2$. To get the value of expected $PaCO_2$ following formula may be applied:

$$\text{Expected PaCO}_2 = \left(0.7.\left[\text{HCO}_3^-\right]\right) + 20 \pm 2\,\text{mmHg} \quad (4.3)$$

  - If, measured $PaCO_2$ > Expected $PaCO_2$ = Additional Respiratory Acidosis.
  - If, measured $PaCO_2$ < Expected $PaCO_2$ = Additional Respiratory Alkalosis.

- **Respiratory Acidosis:** Expected compensatory response for primary respiratory acidosis is an increase in $HCO_3$. As complete compensation may take 2–5 days, the interpretation of metabolic compensation in primary respiratory disorder is little more complicated. In this chapter, we shall follow the approach suggested by Berend and colleagues, as given below [1]:

- For every 10 mm Hg increase in $PaCO_2$ above 40 mm Hg, if $[HCO_3^-]$ increase by 1 mmol/L = Acute Respiratory Acidosis and no second disorder.
- For every 10 mm Hg increase in $PaCO_2$ above 40 mm Hg, if $[HCO_3^-]$ increase by 4–5 mmol/L = Chronic Respiratory Acidosis and no second disorder.
- For every 10 mm Hg increase in $PaCO_2$ above 40 mm Hg, if $[HCO_3^-]$ increase by <1 mmol/L = Additional Metabolic Acidosis.
- For every 10 mm Hg increase in $PaCO_2$ above 40 mm Hg, if $[HCO_3^-]$ increase by >5 mmol/L = Additional Metabolic Alkalosis.

• **Respiratory Alkalosis:** Expected compensatory response in primary respiratory alkalosis is a fall in $[HCO_3^-]$. Complete compensation takes 2–5 days. Formulas for calculating compensatory responses are given below [1].

- For every 10 mm Hg $PaCO_2$ decrease below 40 mm Hg, if $[HCO_3^-]$ decrease by 2 mmol/L = Acute Respiratory Alkalosis and no second disorder.
- For every 10 mm Hg $PaCO_2$ decrease below 40 mm Hg, if $[HCO_3^-]$ decrease by 4–5 mmol/L = Chronic Respiratory Alkalosis and no second disorder.
- For every 10 mm Hg $PaCO_2$ decrease below 40 mm Hg, if $[HCO_3^-]$ decrease by <2 mmol/L = Additional Metabolic Alkalosis.
- For every 10 mm Hg $PaCO_2$ decrease below 40 mm Hg, if $[HCO_3^-]$ decrease by >5 mmol/L = Additional Metabolic Acidosis.

**STEP 4: Look for "ANION GAP"**

• According to the principle of electroneutrality, the sum of cations in any body fluid (including plasma) must be equal to the sum of anions in the fluid. That means:

$$\left[Na^{+}\right]+\left[K^{+}\right]+\text{Unmeasured cations}=\left[Cl^{-}\right]+\left[HCO_3^{-}\right]+\text{Unmeasured anions} \quad (4.4)$$

- To state the equation differently:

$$\text{Unmeasured anions}-\text{Unmeasured cations}=\left[Na^{+}\right]+\left[K^{+}\right]-\left[Cl^{-}\right]-\left[HCO_3^{-}\right] \quad (4.5)$$

- This difference in concentration between plasma unmeasured anions and cations is called "**ANION GAP (AG)**". Since the extracellular concentration of [$K^+$] is low and body needs to maintain its concentration within a narrow range, [$K^+$] can be omitted from this Eq. (4.5). Thus, anion gap can be calculated simply as:

$$\text{Anion Gap}=\left[Na^{+}\right]-\left(\left[Cl^{-}\right]+\left[HCO_3^{-}\right]\right) \quad (4.6)$$

- Normally the gap between unmeasured anions and cations (or anion gap) is filled up mostly by albumin and to a lesser extent by phosphate or lactate. Albumin level is often low in critically ill patients and calculated AG must be corrected for low albumin level.
  - AG can be corrected for albumin by adding 2.5 mmol/L to the calculated AG, for every 1 g/dl decrease in Albumin from its normal value of 4 gm/dl.
  - For example: Calculated AG is 5 mmol/L and Serum Albumin is 2 g/dl. Then, corrected AG: 5+ [(4–2) X 2.5] =10.
- For the purpose of further calculation, we shall take normal value of "ANION GAP" as 12 ± 2 mmol/L.
- Calculation of Anion Gap (AG) helps in:
  - Further elucidating causes of metabolic acidosis into "**High AG**" or "**Normal AG**" metabolic acidosis.

- Presence of high AG may be the sole pointer towards the presence of hidden metabolic acidosis, with multiple opposing acid–base abnormalities normalizing pH, $PaCO_2$ and [$HCO_3$–] as seen in Fig. 4.1.
- Serial measurement of AG helps in following effectiveness of therapy, especially in diabetic ketoacidosis.
- Elevated AG may be the only clue to certain clinical disorders. For example, D-lactate is not routinely measured in clinical laboratories. Presence of high AG in a patient presenting with neurological issues and past history of short bowel syndrome maybe the only pointer towards D-lactic acidosis.
- A low AG or negative AG may be a pointer towards unsuspected hypercalcemia or hypermagnesemia or other heavy metal toxicity. Other reasons for the same may be falsely high serum chloride values in the presence of bromide or iodide.

### *4.2.1 High AG Metabolic Acidosis*

- Further analysis of high AG metabolic acidosis is based on history/physical examination, biochemical test results (including blood glucose, kidney function tests, electrolytes, serum osmolality, toxin levels, etc.).
- An approach to High AG Metabolic acidosis is shown in Fig. 4.2 [1].

### *4.2.2 Normal AG Metabolic Acidosis*

- Further analysis of normal AG metabolic acidosis requires history/physical examination, serum and urinary electrolytes and urine pH.
- An approach to normal AG metabolic acidosis is given in Fig. 4.3 [1].

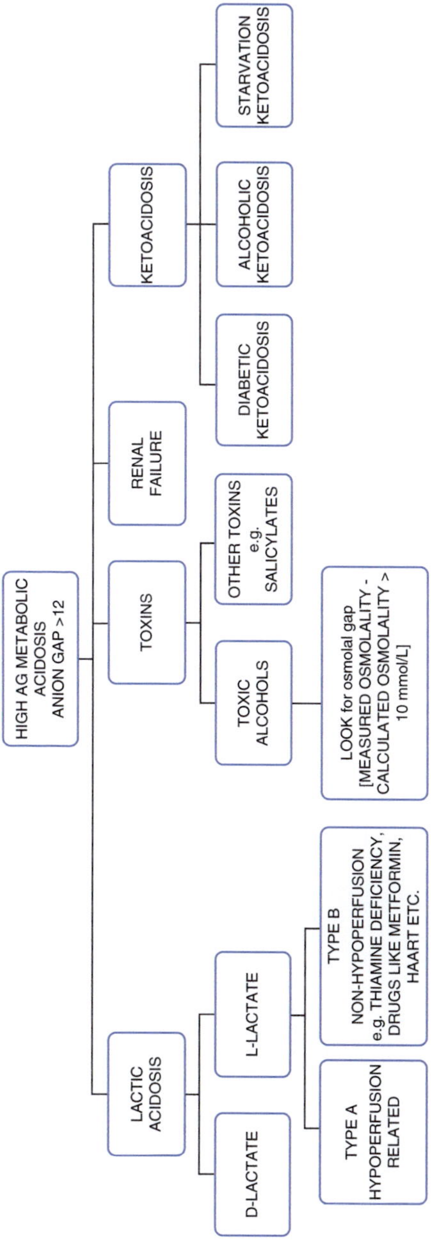


FIGURE 4.2 Approach to high anion gap metabolic acidosis [Adapted from Reference 1]

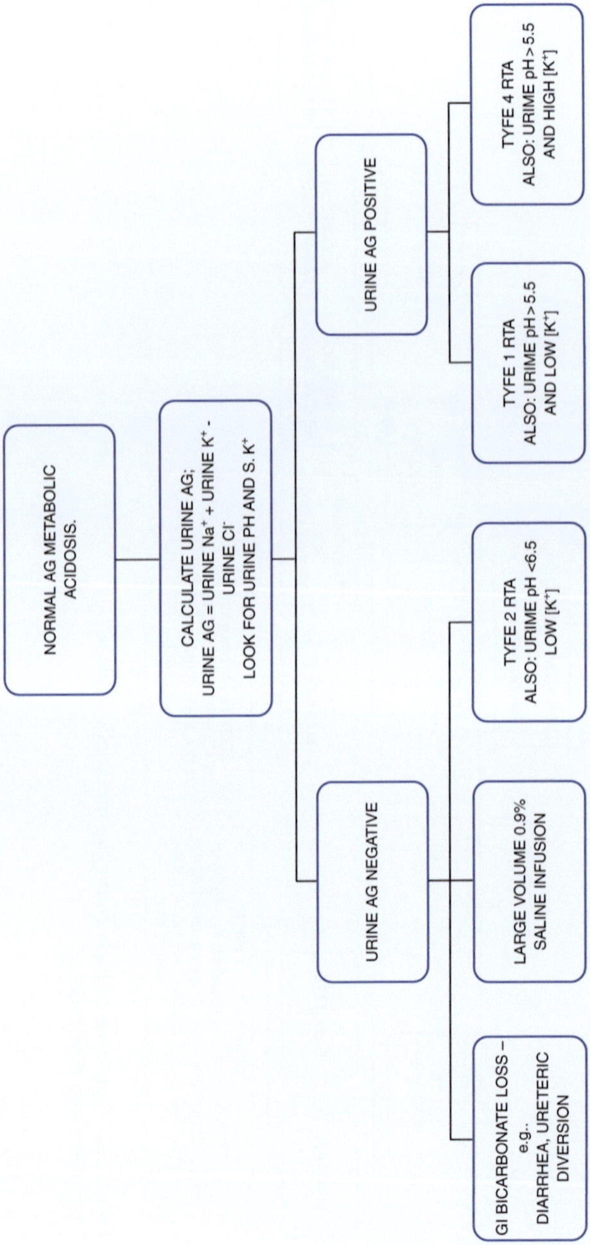


FIGURE 4.3 Approach to normal anion gap metabolic acidosis [Adapted from Reference 1]

**STEP 5: Exploring the Delta Anion Gap—Look for the third disorder**

- The magnitude of increase in anion gap from upper limit of normal (12 mmol/L) (henceforth ΔAG) is closely related to the decrease in [$HCO_3^-$] from normal value of 24.
  - The relationship is 1:1 in case of ketoacidosis. That means, in cases of diabetic ketoacidosis decrease in [$HCO_3^-$] value is expected to be same as decrease in AG from normal [ΔAG].
  - But in cases of lactic acidosis it is 1:0.6. That means, [$HCO_3^-$] value will decrease by 60% of ΔAG.
- This relationship can be explored further by calculating expected [$HCO_3^-$] from ΔAG, to look for the presence of any third disorder.
  - For ketoacidosis or any other high AG acidosis: Expected [$HCO_3^-$] = [24 –. Anion Gap] ± 5.
  - For lactic acidosis: Expected [$HCO_3$–] = [24 – (0.6 ×. Anion Gap)] ± 5.
  - If the actual [$HCO_3^-$] is less than expected [$HCO_3^-$] = Additional normal AG Metabolic Acidosis.
  - If the actual [$HCO_3^-$] is more than expected [$HCO_3^-$] = Additional Metabolic Alkalosis.

**STEP 6: Exploring Metabolic Alkalosis**

- Metabolic Alkalosis is either because of gain of alkali or excess renal retention of [$HCO_3^-$].
- If the effective circulating volume is reduced, renin–angiotensin–aldosterone system is activated and kidneys try to restore volume by re-absorption of filtered [$HCO_3^-$] along with [$Na^+$] and [$Cl^-$], resulting in Metabolic Alkalosis. In these patients, spot urinary [$Cl^-$] concentration is usually <25 mmol/L and pH may be restored by administration of 0.9% Saline (so-called “**Chloride Responsive**”).
- Metabolic alkalosis is also seen in conditions with mineralocorticoid excess (either true or functional) and in patients with [$K^+$] deficiency. In these patients, excretion of [$Na^+$] and [$Cl^-$] in urine is inappropriately high (urinary

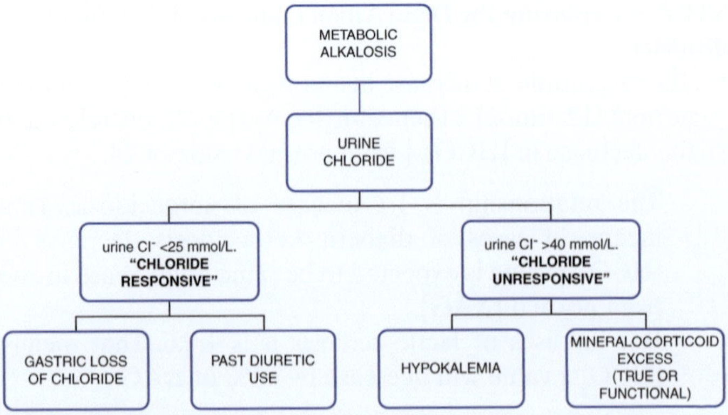


FIGURE 4.4 Approach to metabolic alkalosis [Adapted from Reference 1]

[$Cl^-$] concentration usually >40 mmol/L) and pH is not restored by administration of normal saline (so-called "**Chloride Unresponsive**").

- A suggested approach to metabolic alkalosis is given in Fig. 4.4 [1].

**STEP 7: Exploring the Respiratory Component**

- There are two aspects of the respiratory component.
- First aspect is differentiating between acute and chronic respiratory disorders and is covered in earlier sections (Step 2).
- Second aspect is to make a differentiation between primary pulmonary cause of respiratory component from the extra-pulmonary causes. Calculation of Alveolar-Arterial Oxygen Gradient ($P_{[A\text{-}a]}O_2$) can help in differentiating between these two. If $P_{[A\text{-}a]}O_2$ is >20 mmHg, Respiratory acidosis is due to pulmonary cause.
- $P_{[A\text{-}a]}O_2$ can be calculated from the formula given below. $P_{[A\text{-}a]}O_2$ = $FIO_2$ X (Barometric Pressure [PB] – Water Vapour Pressure [$P_{H2O}$]) –.

$$PaO_2 - \left(PaCO_2 / \text{Gas} - \text{exchange Ratio}\left[R\right]\right) \quad (4.7)$$

- At sea level and a body temperature of 37 °C, the alveolar–arterial difference can be estimated as:

$$FIO_2\,X(760-47)-PaO_2-(PaCO_2/0.8)$$
$$[PB=760\,mmHg, P_{H2O}=47\,mmHg, R=0.8] \quad (4.8)$$

- Figure 4.5 provides some clinical examples of respiratory acid–base disorders and how they can be differentiated from each other using the approach described above [1].

## 4.3 Limitations of Traditional Approach

- There are several strengths of traditional approach including its apparent simplicity, wide acceptability and its ability to identify a vast majority of acid–base abnormalities in clinical medicine. But there are several limitations of this approach and it fails to answer many pertinent questions.
  - It does not tell us about the mechanism of metabolic changes. How can $[H^+]$ with a tiny plasma concentration (40 nmol/L at physiological pH of 7.4 and 38 ° C temperature, compared to $[H_2O]$ in 55.3 mol/L and $[Na^+]$ in 140 mmol/L) directly manipulates the plasma pH?
  - Its presumption of $[HCO_3^-]$ independent variable determining metabolic component of acid–base balance is irrational, when it is in equilibrium with $CO_2$.
  - It does not tell us about the role of buffer bases other than $[PaCO_2/HCO_3^-]$.
  - It fails to give the clinician magnitude of changes in the metabolic component.

## 4.4 Stewart's Physicochemical Approach

- In the late 1970s, Peter Stewart, a Canadian biophysicist, described a quantitative approach to acid–base disorder [2]. His approach is based on fundamental physicochemical properties of a solution and includes principles of elec-

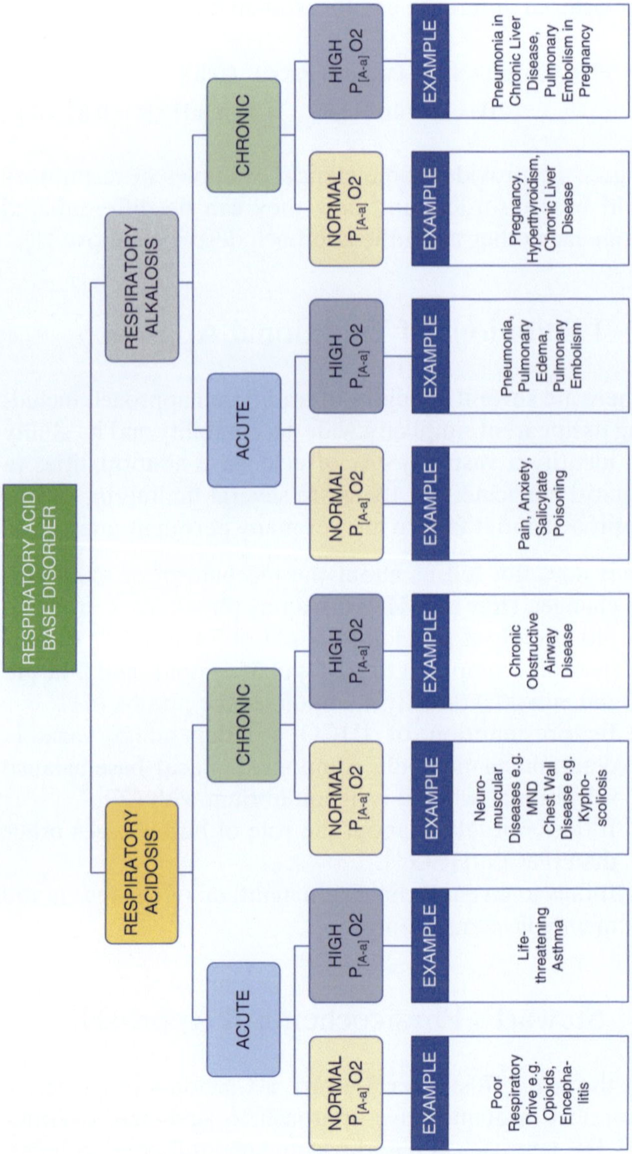


FIGURE 4.5 Approach to respiratory acid–base disorders

troneutrality, law of conservation of mass and dissociation equilibrium of all incompletely dissociated substances in a solution.

- Stewart approach emphasizes that [$HCO_3-$] and pH in body fluids are dependent variables and are determined by three independent variables:
  - *Strong Ion difference (SID).*
  - *Concentration of weak non-volatile acids (Atot).* Mostly determined by Albumin concentration or phosphate.
  - *Total CO2 content* (this incorporates $PaCO_2$, $H_2CO_3$ and $HCO_3$).
- Stewart concept simply states that any changes in these three independent variables, distort the dissociation equilibrium of weakly dissociating substances in plasma (including water itself) altering the balance between [$H^+$] and [$OH^-$]. *Relative increase or decrease in [H+] (compared to [OH−]) produces acidosis and alkalosis, respectively (Arrhenius definition of acid/base).*

## 4.4.1 Strong Ion Difference (SID)

- Strong ions are derived from substances that are almost completely dissociated in a solution. The strong ion difference (SID) is the sum of routinely measured strong plasma cations ([$Na^+$], [$K^+$], [$Ca^{2+}$], [$Mg^{2+}$]) minus the routinely measured strong plasma anions (mostly [$Cl^-$]) (also called "**Apparent SID**" by some authors [3]).
  - Calculation of apparent SID does not take into consideration "Unmeasured Strong Anions" that are present only in miniscule concentrations in a physiological state.

$$\text{Apparent SID} = \left(\left[Na^+\right]+\left[K^+\right]+\left[Ca^{2+}\right]+\left[Mg^{2+}\right]\right)-\left(\left[Cl^-\right]\right) \tag{4.9}$$

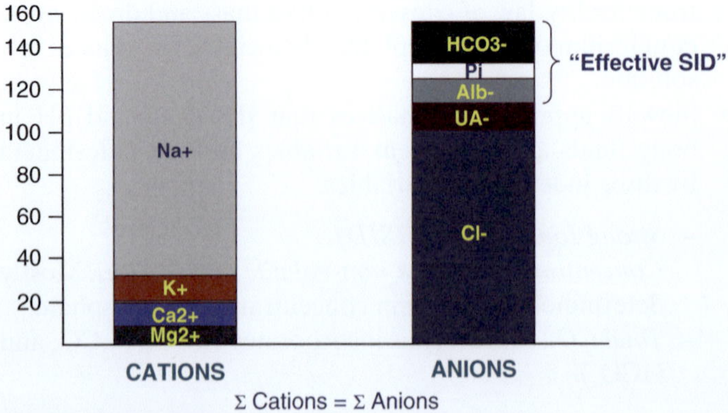


FIGURE 4.6 Gamblegram showing principle of electroneutrality and concept of SID

- This concept can be understood pictorially from the Gamblegram shown in Fig. 4.5 depicting the concept of electroneutrality.
- From Fig. 4.6, we can see that the gap between strong cations ([$Na^+$], [$K^+$], [$Ca^{2+}$], [$Mg^{2+}$]) and strong anions([$Cl^-$]) (or apparent SID), is filled up mostly by [$HCO_3^-$] and total amount of non-volatile acids anions ([Atot] comprising mostly of [$Alb^-$] and to a lesser extent [$Pi^-$]).
  - Thus, SID can also be calculated alternatively as the sum of [$HCO_3^-$] and [Atot] (also called "**Effective SID**" by some authors [3]).

$$\text{Effective SID} = \left[HCO_3^-\right] + \left[Alb^-\right] + \left[Pi^-\right] \tag{4.10}$$

  - If the "Apparent SID" and "Effective SID" do not match (a condition Kellum referred to as "**Strong Ion Gap or SIG**"), it signifies the presence of unmeasured strong anions.

$$\text{SIG} = \text{Apparent SID} - \text{Effective SID} \tag{4.11}$$

- SID can decrease with any gain in unmeasured strong anions (e.g. beta-hydroxybutyrate or lactate) without an equivalent increase in strong cations. Alternatively, a decrease in SID can simply be because of [$Cl^-$] and [$Na^+$] moving closer together, either because of water excess (lowering [$Na^+$]) or because of an increase in [$Cl^-$].
  - Decrease in SID results in metabolic acidosis.
  - From Fig. 4.5, it can be seen that a decrease in SID in turn decreases the available space between strong cations and strong anions, resulting in a decrease in [$HCO_3^-$] (see Fig. 4.5).
  - *Thus, the low [HCO3−] seen in metabolic acidosis is the effect (or marker) of metabolic acidosis rather than its cause.*
- On the other hand, an increase in SID results in metabolic alkalosis.
  - SID can either increase as a result of an increase in [$Na^+$] (reflecting water deficit) or because of a decrease in [$Cl^-$].
  - With more available space, [$HCO_3^-$] increases with an increase in [SID].

### *4.4.2 Total Non-Volatile Acid Anion ($A_{TOT}$)*

- An increase [Atot] can result in metabolic acidosis and decrease in [$HCO_3^-$] (with unchanged SID).
- Similarly, decrease in [Atot] (commonly due to hypoalbuminemia in critically ill) results in metabolic alkalosis and increase in [$HCO_3^-$].

### *4.4.3 Total $CO_2$*

- Stewart gave the concept of total $CO_2$ (that incorporates $PaCO_2$, $H_2CO_3$ and [$HCO_3^-$]) in regulating pH.

- This concept gives importance to $H_2CO_3$ and $[HCO_3^-]$ in acid–base physiology but emphasizes that neither $H_2CO3$ nor $[HCO_3^-]$ can independently regulate acid–base balance, as long as there is sufficient carbonic anhydrase (an enzyme that modifies the reaction between $H_2O$ and $CO_2$ generating $HCO_3^-$ and $H^+$), an intact circulation (that carries $CO_2$ from tissue to lung) and normal functioning lungs (that regulate $PaCO_2$).

### *4.4.4 Stewart at Bedside*

- At the bedside, the concept can be applied simply from routine blood gas and biochemical measurements as shown in Fig. 4.7.
- Since strong ions like $[K^+]$, $[Ca^{2+}]$ and $[Mg^{2+}]$ are tightly regulated and changes very little in normal physiological state, [SID] is mostly determined by $[Na^+]$ and $[Cl^-]$ concentration in plasma.

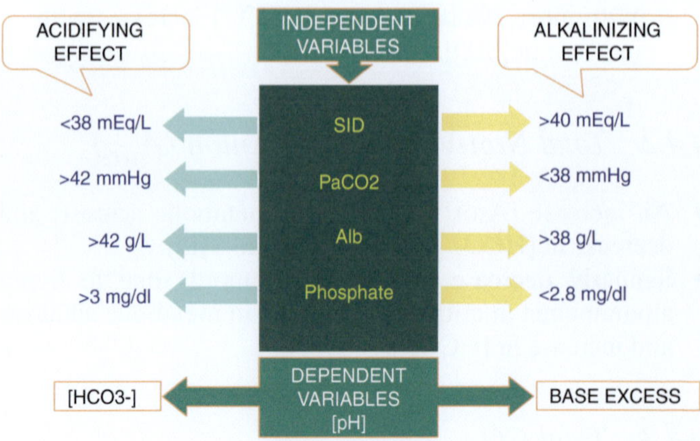


FIGURE 4.7 Overview of Stewart's concept

### 4.4.5 *Quantifying Stewart: Fencl–Leith Modification*

- In 1993, Fencl and Leith proposed a simplified approach to Stewart's physicochemical concept by quantifying values of independent variables [4]. This modified approach provides an insight into the mechanism of acid–base abnormality and use the same for providing a management plan.
  - Acid–base status of the plasma can be considered normal only when all independent variables are within normal range. In contrast abnormality of any one of these independent variables lead to acid–base disturbances.
- Values for all independent variables can either be obtained directly or may be easily calculated from the arterial blood gas analyzer and routine biochemistry.
  - **PaCO2:** Obtained from the blood gas machine.
  - **Water excess/deficit:** Any deviation in $[Na^+]$ (Normal value $[Na^+] = 140 \pm 2$ mEq/L), low value signifying water deficit and high-value water excess.
  - **[Cl−] excess or deficit:** Normal value is $[Cl^-]$ is taken as 102 mEq/L for further calculation. Observed $[Cl^-]$ value needs correction for any dilution/ concentration of plasma. This can be done by the following equation:

$$\left[Cl^-\right]_{Corrected} = \left[Cl^-\right]_{Observed} \times \left(\left[Na^+\right]_{Normal} \div \left[Na^+\right]_{Observed}\right) \tag{4.12}$$

$$\text{Chloride Excess/deficit} = [Cl^-]_{Normal} - [Cl^-]_{Corrected}$$

  - **SID:** SID in plasma can be derived as the sum of [HCO-] plus the negative electric charges contributed by albumin [Alb-] and by inorganic phosphate [Pi-]. $[HCO_3^-]$ is available from arterial blood gas machine or routine biochemistry values. [Alb-] and [Pi-] (in mEq/L) can be calculated from the measured Albumin (in gm/L), [Pi] (mmol/L), as per equations proposed by Fencl and colleagues [5] and modified by Story and colleagues [6] Normal value of SID is taken as 39∓1 mEq/L for further calculation.

$$[\text{Alb}-] = 0.25 \times \text{Alb}(\text{in g/L}) \tag{4.13}$$

$$[\text{Pi}-] = 0.6 \times \text{Phosphate}(\text{in mg/dl}) \tag{4.14}$$

$$\text{SID} = \left[\text{HCO}_3^-\right] + \left[\text{Alb}^-\right] + \left[\text{Pi}^-\right] \tag{4.15}$$

– **Unidentified strong anions [UA-]:** [UA-] are strong anions other than Cl– (included in the differential diagnosis of high Anion Gap metabolic acidosis e.g. lactate, keto-acids and other organic anions, sulphate). Normal range for [UA-] is taken as 8 ∓ 2 mEq/L. Value of [UA-] can be indirectly derived from the equation below:

$$\begin{aligned}\text{Unmeasured Anion} = {} & \left[\text{Na}^+\right] + \left[\text{K}^+\right] + \left[\text{Ca}^{2+}\right] + \left[\text{Mg}^{2+}\right] \\ & - \left[\text{Cl}^-\right] - [\text{SID}]\end{aligned} \tag{4.16}$$

(For routine purpose [$Mg^{2+}$] may be replaced by 1.7)

Once these values are obtained, acid–base status of the patient can be classified into the classification schema given in Table 4.1.

## 4.5 Case Scenario (Continued)

- With normal pH, PaCO2, Base Excess and corrected Anion Gap (9.75) values, Mr. MJ apparently does not have any acid–base disorder (following Traditional approach).

TABLE 4.1 Classification of acid–base disturbances

| | Acidosis | Alkalosis |
|---|---|---|
| Respiratory | ↑ $PaCO_2$ | ↓ $PaCO_2$ |
| *Metabolic* | | |
| Abnormal SID | | |
| 1. Water excess/deficit. | ↓ $[Na^+]$ | ↑ $[Na^+]$ |
| 2. Imbalance of strong anions. | | |
| – Chloride excess/deficit. | ↑ $[cl^-]$ | ↓ $[cl^-]$ |
| – Unidentified anion ([XA-]) excess. | ↑ [XA-] | – |
| Non-volatile weak acids | | |
| 1. Serum albumin. | ↑ $[Alb^-]$ | ↓ $[Alb^-]$ |
| 2. Inorganic phosphate. | ↑ $[pi^-]$ | ↓ $[pi^-]$ |

But that seems to be unusual considering the overall clinical status of the patient!

- Applying Fencl–Stewart approach, he has:
  - No respiratory abnormality (PaCO2 39 mmHg)
  - Low sodium: 129 mEq/L suggesting water excess
  - High $[Cl-]_{Corrected}$: 98 × (142/125) = 111 mEq/L
  - Low SID ($[HCO_3^-]$ + [Alb−] + [Pi−]): 24 + 3.25 + 0.9 = 28.15 mEq/L (Albuminate: 0.25 × 13 = 3.25 mEq/L
  - Pi: 0.6 × 1.5 = 0.9 mEq/L)
  - Unmeasured anion within normal range: ([Na+] + [K+] + [Ca2+] + [Mg2+] − [Cl−] − [SID]) ~0 mEq/L (within normal range)
- Thus, from Stewart's Physicochemical Approach, one can easily find that Mr. MJ has multiple acid–base abnormalities including low SID metabolic acidosis (related to both water excess and high corrected chloride) and metabolic alkalosis (related to low Albumin value).

**Take-Home Messages**

- Traditional approach to acid–base disturbances is widely used and has the ability to resolve most clinical problems.
- However, it fails to provide insight into the pathogenesis of complex disorders.
- Stewart's approach can provide insight into the pathogenesis of acid–base abnormalities, help in identifying hidden acid–base disorder, quantify individual components of complex acid–base abnormalities and provide the clinician an approach to decide probable ways to rectify the problem (if necessary).
- Understanding Stewart's approach to acid–base abnormalities will be very useful to understand the effects of different intravenous fluids on acid–base physiology of plasma, as will be discussed in subsequent chapters.

## References

1. Berend K, de Vries APJ, Gans ROB. Physiological approach to assessment of acid–base disturbances. N Engl J Med. 2014;371:1434–45.
2. Stewart PA. How to understand acid-base. A qualitative acid-base primer for biology and medicine. New York: Elsevier North Holland Inc; 1981.
3. Kellum JA. Determinants of blood pH in health and disease. Crit Care. 2000;4:6.
4. Fencl V, Leith DE. Stewart's quantitative acid–base chemistry: applications in biology and medicine. Respir Physiol. 1993;91:1–16.
5. Fencl V, Jabor A, Kazda A, Figge J. Diagnosis of metabolic acid–base disturbances in critically ill patients. Am J Respir Crit Care Med. 2000;162:2246–51.
6. Story DA, Morimatsu H, Bellomo R. Strong ions, weak acids and base excess: a simplified Fencl-Stewart approach to clinical acid-base disorders. Br J Anaesth. 2004;92:54–60.

# Part II
# Fluid Types and Vasopressors

# Chapter 5
# Crystalloids as Resuscitation Fluid

## 5.1 Case Scenario 1

Mr. AA, a 74-year-old gentleman with past history of diabetes mellitus and nephropathy presented to the ED with 3-days history of fever, cough and progressive breathlessness. On examination, he was confused, febrile with a regular heart rate of 112/min, blood pressure of 84/46 mmHg, respiratory rate of 30/min and $SpO_2$ of 96% on 4 litres of $O_2$ by nasal prong. Lung auscultation revealed bronchial breathing in left infrascapular and left axillary region suggestive of consolidation. Arterial blood gas showed pH 7.36, $PaO_2$ 64 mmHg, $PaCO_2$ 32.8 mmHg, $HCO_3^-$ 19.2 mmol/L and lactate 4.6 mmol/L. ED physician was aware of the latest surviving sepsis guideline recommending rapid intravenous crystalloid bolus for initial resuscitation of Mr. AA.

## 5.2 Case Scenario 2

Ms. GA, a 28-year-old female was brought to the ED following a road traffic accident. On examination, her Glasgow Coma Scale was E1M4V2 and she was moving all four limbs.



S. Ghosh, *Handbook of Intravenous Fluids*,
https://doi.org/10.1007/978-981-19-0500-1_5

Her pupils were equal in size and were reacting to light. She had a heart rate of 112/min and blood pressure of 80/40 mmHg. Her breathing pattern was visibly laboured with bilateral equal breath sound on auscultation of chest. Her abdomen was distended. She also had a swollen left thigh, possibly haematoma. She was intubated and connected with ventilator. It was also decided to give her a bolus of warm intravenous crystalloid while waiting for blood products.

### *5.2.1 How to Choose the Most Appropriate Crystalloid for Resuscitating an Individual Patient?*

Administration of rapid intravenous fluid bolus with an aim to quickly restore the intravascular volume is one of the commonest (and favourite) practices in an acute care setting. The physiological rationale and limitations of fluid resuscitation are already discussed in Chap. 1. In this chapter and in Chap. 6, I shall be discussing different formulations used for resuscitation, their relative advantages and disadvantages. I shall also be providing ready recommendations for bedside practice at the end of each chapter.

## 5.3 Resuscitation Fluids

- "**Resuscitation Fluids**" can be pragmatically defined as any intravenous fluid formulation rapidly administered at a rate of more than 500 ml/hour to quickly restore circulation in shock state.
  - Ideally, a resuscitation fluid should have the ability to increase intravascular volume in a predictable and sustained manner, should have a composition closer to extracellular fluid including their electrolyte contents and tonicity, should be metabolizable and excreted completely without accumulation in the tissues, should not be having any systemic adverse effects and should

be widely available and cost-effective. Unfortunately, no such ideal fluid exists in the real world.

- Resuscitation fluids are broadly classified into crystalloids and colloids.
  - *Crystalloids are intravenous fluid formulations that contain glucose and/or salt in clear solution (***e.g.** *0.9% saline, Ringer's lactate, etc.).* Besides resuscitation, crystalloids solutions are also used for replacing ongoing fluid loss due to diarrhoea or vomiting or nasogastric suctioning ("**Replacement Fluid**" discussed briefly in Chap. 13) or for maintaining hydration of patients who are unable to drink ("**Maintenance Fluid**", discussed in Chap. 7) and also as vehicles for the delivery of drugs.
  - *Colloids can be defined as fluid formulations that contain microscopic particles (***e.g.** *starch, dextran or albumin) suspended in some crystalloid solution (***e.g.** *6% hydroxyethyl starch, 20% albumin, etc.).* Colloid formulations will be discussed in Chap. 6.

## 5.4 Crystalloid Resuscitation

- Choice of crystalloids for resuscitation is based on the composition of different formulations, sodium and chloride content, strong ion difference (SID), tonicity, availability and cost. Perhaps a more important factor is the clinician's familiarity with specific formulation.
- To be effective, a significant proportion of resuscitation fluid infused must remain in the intravascular compartment. That is why only isotonic or hypertonic fluids are effective for the purpose of resuscitation, as hypotonic fluids will be distributed quickly to the intracellular and interstitial compartment from the intravascular compartment.
- Electrolyte contents, SID and osmolality of commonly used crystalloid formulations for resuscitation are given in Table 5.1.

TABLE 5.1 Composition of crystalloid resuscitation fluids and their comparison with human plasma

| | Plasma | 0.9% saline | Ringer lactate | Plasmalyte | Sterofundin |
|---|---|---|---|---|---|
| Na (mmol/L) | 136–145 | 154 | 129 | 140 | 145 |
| K (mmol/L) | 3.5–5 | | 5 | 5 | 4 |
| Ca (mmol/L) | 2.2–2.6 | | 2.5 | | 2.5 |
| Mg (mmol/L) | 0.8–1 | | | 1.5 | 1 |
| Cl (mmol/L) | 98–106 | 154 | 109 | 98 | 127 |
| Acetate (mmol/L) | | | | 27 | 24 |
| Gluconate (mmol/L) | | | | 23 | |
| Lactate (mmol/L) | <1 | | 29 | | |
| Maleate (mmol/L) | | | | | 5 |
| SID (mEq/L) | 40 | 0 | 27 | 50 | 25.5 |
| Calculated osmolality (mOsmol/L) | 285–295 | 308 | 273 | 295 | 304 |
| Effective osmolality (mOsmol/L) | 285–295 | 286 | 254 | 270 | 290 |

## 5.5 Isotonic Saline or 0.9% Saline

- The exact origin of isotonic saline is not known. Perhaps it is related to the in vitro experiment by Dr. Hamburger (of "Hamburger shift of Chloride Shift" fame) on red blood cell lysis in different concentrations of sodium chloride solution conducted in the 1880s. He demonstrated that

RBCs do not lyse when suspended in sodium chloride concentration of 0.9% and somewhat erroneously suggested that sodium chloride concentration in human blood is 0.9%. This is probably the origin of "Normal" being attached to 0.9% saline solution. We now know that the salt concentration in human blood is 0.6% (not 0.9%). Here are some useful facts about 0.9% Saline:

- Isotonic saline is the most commonly used fluid worldwide.
- Despite being known as "normal", it has virtually no similarity with plasma in terms of composition and physiological properties (Table 5.1).
- Compared to plasma, it has much higher sodium and chloride content, absence of electrolytes except Na and Cl, a SID of 0 and higher calculated osmolality.
- Interestingly, effective osmolality of isotonic saline in body temperature is 286 mOsmol/L making it isotonic to human plasma in vivo.

- **Advantages of Isotonic Saline:**
  - Widely available and familiar intravenous formulation
  - Cheap
  - Can be used in patients with raised intracranial pressure (Isotonic to human plasma)
  - Compatible with blood, blood products and many other medications (as diluent)
- **Disadvantages of Isotonic Saline:**
  - Because of high chloride content and SID of 0, 0.9% Saline is associated with a high risk of hyperchloremic metabolic acidosis, especially when infused in large volumes. Hyperchloremia may be associated with decreased renal blood flow and acute renal injury (discussed in subsequent section) [1].
  - High volume of isotonic saline infusion is also associated with endothelial damage (glycocalyx damage), gastrointestinal dysfunction (related to gut edema) and coagulopathy, in experimental studies.

### *5.5.1 Hyperchloremia and Renal Injury*

- Large volume of sodium and chloride-rich fluid infusion results in high glomerular filtration of both sodium and chloride. We know from our physiology knowledge that high-sodium and chloride content near macula densa (as a consequence of high glomerular filtration) causes vasoconstriction of afferent arteriole (also known as "**Tubuloglomerular Feedback**" as can be seen in Fig. 5.1).
  - Afferent arteriolar constriction from tubuloglomerular feedback leads to a decrease in glomerular perfusion,

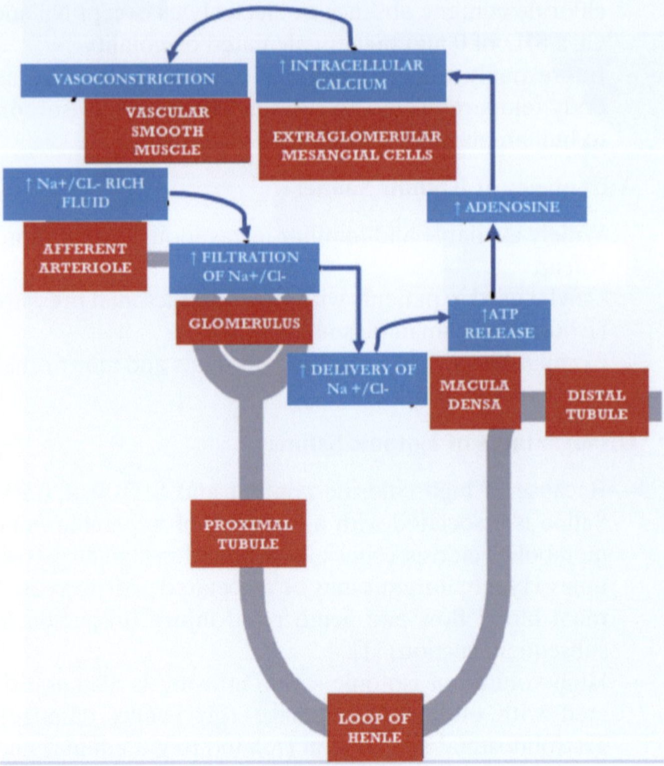


FIGURE 5.1 Tubuloglomerular feedback

decreased glomerular filtration and may potentially result in worsening of renal function.

- Worsening of renal function by infusion of fluids with high chloride content has been demonstrated in animal and human volunteer studies [1].
  - However, in an acute care setting, many questions still remain unanswered. Is there any subgroup of patients more susceptible to this adverse renal outcome? Is there any cut-off concentration of chloride and volume of infusion of 0.9% Saline at which this adverse renal outcome is more common?

### 5.5.2 *Balanced Crystalloids*

- Balanced formulations are crystalloids containing electrolytes in a concentration closer to plasma (e.g. Ringer's lactate, Plasmalyte, Sterofundin, etc.).
- They all have less chloride content compared to 0.9% saline and to maintain electroneutrality they contain different metabolizable organic anions, e.g. lactate, acetate, maleate or gluconate. Rapid metabolism of these organic anions results in an increase in SID of balanced solutions in vivo.
- In subsequent paragraphs, we shall discuss "**10 interesting facts**" one should know about balanced fluids:
  1. Although the chloride concentration of balanced solutions is closer to plasma, they are neither perfect nor physiological. Organic anions present in these solutions are much higher than that of plasma e.g. lactate concentration in Ringer's lactate is almost 30 times that of plasma. Presence of acetate, gluconate or maleate is almost negligible in human plasma.
  2. Although different buffered solutions are clubbed together under a single umbrella term "Balanced Fluids" they are not biologically equivalent. The concentration of ancillary cations (e.g. sodium, potassium, calcium, magnesium) is variable in different solutions, as can be

seen in Table 5.1. Moreover, they have significant differences in buffering substances present in them.

3. Ringer's Lactate and Ringer's Acetate are relatively hypotonic compared to plasma. Plasmalyte also has low effective osmolality (in vivo). Hypotonic solutions may potentially increase brain edema especially in the setting of disrupted blood–brain barrier. Hence, they should be used with caution during resuscitation of a patient with traumatic brain injury or in any other patient at a risk of raised intracranial pressure [2].
4. SID of balanced solutions is different (29 mEq/l for Ringer's lactate compared to 50 mEq/l for Plasmalyte) producing variable effects on acid–base balance. As a rule of thumb, if the SID of a particular solution is lower than the measured plasma bicarbonate [$HCO_3^-$], infusion of a large volume of that solution will produce metabolic acidosis and vice versa [3].

- For example, large volume of 0.9% Saline (with SID of 0) will produce metabolic acidosis if the baseline plasma [$HCO_3^-$] is 24 mmol/L (or any values above 0).
- If the baseline plasma [$HCO_3^-$] is 24 mmol/L, infusion of large volume RL (with SID of 27) will produce metabolic alkalosis.

5. Lactate is metabolized primarily in liver and metabolism of lactate may be overwhelmed in the presence of severe hepatic dysfunction. There is also a theoretical risk of high lactate content in Ringer's solution, interfering with measured lactate value, used for monitoring resuscitation. But the later concern has not been substantiated in clinical studies.
6. Compared to lactate, the metabolism of acetate is less dependent on hepatic function. However, in animal studies, a high level of acetate had shown to produce myocardial toxicity and hypotension. Fortunately, similar findings have not been demonstrated in human studies so far.
7. Gluconate is metabolized very slowly and almost excreted unchanged in urine. This slow metabolism of

gluconate reduces the SID of Plasmalyte when measured in vivo and keeps it closer to physiological range. Interestingly gluconate in Plasmalyte can give a false-positive result for galactomannan assay used for invasive mold infection.

8. Little is known about maleate metabolism.
9. There is a theoretical risk of potentiating hyperkalemia by infusion of K+ containing balanced solutions, especially in patients with borderline or high serum potassium levels or in patients at a higher risk of hyperkalemia (e.g. chronic kidney disease).

- However, this theoretical concern has not been substantiated in clinical studies. In fact, controlled trials (Table 5.2) have shown a higher risk of hyperkalemia with 0.9% saline infusion compared to balanced fluid.
- There are two plausible explanations for balanced fluid not producing hyperkalemia. (a) Rapid dilution of $K^+$ content of balanced fluids in the large extracellular fluid compartment. (b) High SID of balanced salt solutions alkalinizing the extracellular and moving $K^+$ to the intracellular compartment.

10. There is a theoretical concern about infusion of calcium-containing balanced salt solutions (Ringer's Lactate and Sterofundin) along with blood transfusion and possible precipitation of citrate leading to clot formation. However, this concern again has not been substantiated in clinical studies.

## 5.6 0.9% Saline Versus Balanced Salt Solutions

- There is enough physiological rationale in favour of using balanced fluids over 0.9% Saline in most clinical scenarios as discussed above. Large observational studies have also demonstrated several advantages of balanced fluids for resuscitation including favourable effects on mortality and renal outcome [7–9].

- However, these obvious advantages of balanced fluid solutions have not yet been unequivocally substantiated in randomized trials till date. Table 5.3 summarizes data from RCTs comparing saline and balanced solutions.

TABLE 5.2 Results of clinical trials comparing 0.9% saline versus balanced salt solution

| | **O'Malley et al.** [4] | **Khajavi et al.** [5] | **Modi et al.** [6] |
|---|---|---|---|
| Setting | Single US centre | Single Centre. Iran. | Single Centre. Ahmedabad, India. |
| No of patients | 51 patients | 52 patients | 74 patients |
| Patient group | Intra-operative fluid during kidney transplant. | Intra-operative fluid during kidney transplant. | Intra-operative fluid during kidney transplant. |
| Intervention | 0.9% saline | 0.9% saline | 0.9% saline. |
| Control | Ringer's lactate | Ringer's lactate | Ringer's lactate |
| Primary outcome | No difference in 2 groups in terms of rise in creatinine at Day-3 | No difference in mean creatinine level at Day-3 | pH decreased from 7.43 to 7.33 in saline group. No change in RL group. |
| Secondary outcome | 19% in saline group had $K^+ > 6$ (vs. 0% in RL) 31% in saline group treated for metabolic acidosis (vs 0% in RL) | Lower mean pH in saline group. Higher mean $K^+$ in saline group (4.88 vs 4.03) | Significantly higher $K^+$ level in saline group. |

TABLE 5.3 Randomized studies comparing 0.9% saline versus balanced crystalloids

| | **SPLIT** [10] | **SALT** [11] | **SMART** [12] | **SALT-ED** [13] | **BaSICS** [14] |
|---|---|---|---|---|---|
| Setting | 4-ICUs. Australia and New Zealand | Single Centre in US | Single Centre in US. 5-ICUs | Single Centre in US | 75-ICUs in Brazil |
| No of patients | 2278 | 974 | 15,802 | 13,347 | 11,052 |
| Patient group | Patients requiring IV crystalloid for resuscitation or maintenance | Patients requiring resuscitation with IV crystalloid during ICU stay | Patients requiring resuscitation with IV crystalloid during ICU stay | Patients receiving IV crystalloids >500 ml for resuscitation in ED and admitted to wards. | ICU patients at a high risk of AKI (age > 65, MAP <65 or SBP <90 mmHg, sepsis, on MV, oliguric with creatinine >1.2 mg/dl), requiring fluid expansion. |
| Intervention | Plasmalyte | Any balanced crystalloid | Any balanced crystalloid | Any balanced crystalloid | Plasmalyte |

(continued)

TABLE 5.3 (continued)

| | **SPLIT** [10] | **SALT** [11] | **SMART** [12] | **SALT-ED** [13] | **BaSICS** [14] |
|---|---|---|---|---|---|
| Control | 0.9% saline | 0.9% saline | 0.9% saline | 0.9% saline | 0.9% saline |
| Primary outcome | – No difference in AKI incidence at 90 days. | – 0.9% saline made up a larger proportion of the isotonic crystalloid in saline group than in balanced group | – Incidence of MAKE-30, significantly lower in balanced group. | – Lower hospital free days in balanced group. | – No difference in 90-day mortality. |
| Secondary outcome | – No difference in RRT utilization.<br>– No difference in ICU or hospital mortality. | – No difference in MAKE-30. | – Lower in-hospital mortality at 30-days.<br>– Lower need for new RRT in balanced group.<br>– No difference in persistent renal dysfunction. | – No difference in MAKE-30.<br>– No difference in in-hospital mortality.<br>– No difference in KADIGO stage 2 or higher AKI. | – No difference in renal outcome including need for RRT between groups.<br>– No difference in overall SOFA score at day 7 between groups.<br>– However, there was worse neurological SOFA score at day 7 in intervention group. |

| | | | | |
|---|---|---|---|---|
| Comments | – Predominantly post-operative patients. Only 4% with sepsis. Another 4% with trauma.<br>– Not really sick patients (median APACHE II score ~ 14).<br>– Low median fluid volume ~ 2000 ml (mostly in first 24 hours), making a difference in outcomes potentially less likely.<br>– Resuscitation and maintenance fluid not specified. | – Pilot study to look for feasibility of a larger trial. | – Both SMART and SALT-ED studies are criticized for being single centre, non-blinded trials.<br>– Patient population was not so sick with low overall mortality. Less than 15% of patients had sepsis in SMART.<br>– RL and Plasmalyte (predominantly RL) clubbed together.<br>– Low fluid volume. Median volume from ICU admission to hospital discharge in SMART: ~1000 ml. Median volume ED admission to wards in SALT-ED: ~1000 ml.<br>– MAKE30 as an outcome measure with similar weightage given to death, RRT and persistent renal dysfunction is criticized for not being a true patient-centred outcome. | – 50% elective surgical patients.<br>– Not really sick ICU patients (median APACHE II score 12, SOFA score 4). 40% of patients not hypotensive.<br>– Median volumes of trial fluid administered were low (mean < 1 L/day) making a difference in outcomes potentially less likely.<br>– Administration of non-study fluids in large number of patients might have confounded results. Following randomisation ~30% of the total fluid received by day 3 was non-study crystalloids. |

*MAKE-30* major adverse kidney events at 30-days—a composite of death, new receipt of renal-replacement therapy or persistent renal dysfunction—all censored at hospital discharge or 30 days after enrolment whichever came first, *RRT* renal replacement therapy, *KDIGO* kidney disease improving global outcomes, *RL* Ringer's lactate

- Also, no study has compared so far between different balanced solutions.

- To summarize, expecting any meaningful long-term outcome benefit of any single intervention like fluid resuscitation from randomized clinical trial is perhaps unrealistic, unless a large number of really sick and high-risk patients are included in it (limitations seen in all RCTs done so far).
  - Until then, it is possibly safe to base our practice on strong physiological rationale and observational study data.
  - If available, balanced solutions should be preferred as resuscitation fluid of choice unless contraindicated. However, as of today, there is no clarity on the choice amongst different balanced fluid formulations.
  - 0.9% Saline should be considered in specific circumstances like patients at a higher risk of raised intracranial pressure or hypovolemic patients with metabolic alkalosis (e.g. following profound vomiting).

### *5.6.1 Hypertonic Saline*

- Hypertonic saline solutions are crystalloid intravenous fluids with high concentrations of NaCl dissolved in water. Commonly used preparations include 2%, 3%, 5%, 7% and 23% NaCl. *Among them, only 3% of Saline is commercially available in India.* These solutions are routinely used for treating symptomatic hyponatremia and raised intracranial pressure.
- Besides these two indications, Hypertonic saline solutions are also being used for resuscitation purposes for over three decades.
- The proponents of these solutions claim several potential advantages of them including reduction of the overall infusion volume (expansion of intravascular volume by shifting fluid from extra-vascular space in intact circulation) and favourable effects reported on myocardial contractil-

ity, vascular tone and inflammatory processes in experimental studies.

- However, in patients with renal dysfunction with impaired excretion of saline or with increased vascular permeability (both common scenarios in ICUs), situation may be different. In fact, in the largest clinical trial comparing hypertonic saline with 0.9% saline for resuscitating patients with septic shock, hypertonic saline failed to show any advantage over the comparator (See Box 5.1) [15].

**Box 5.1 "HYPERS2S" Study** [15]

**Research Question:** Is resuscitation with HTS associated with volume sparing?

**Setting:** 22 Centres from France participated in the trial. Double-blind randomized control trial.

**Patient:** 334 Patients with Septic shock on mechanical ventilation and who required volume resuscitation in the first 72 hours after randomization were included in the study.

**Intervention:** 280 ml boluses of 3% Saline in initial 72 Hours.

**Control:** 280 ml boluses of 0.9% Saline in initial 72 Hours.

**Outcome:**

- The study was stopped early because of lack of benefit in the intervention arm and potential harm seen in the other arm of the study that compared hyperoxia with normoxia.
- 28-Day mortality: HTS 42% vs NS 37% (NS)
- No difference in Vasopressor free days, MV free days, RRT free days on Day 29.
- No difference in cumulative volume of resuscitation fluid at 72 hours.

## 5.7 Case Scenarios (Continued)

- In case scenario 1, Mr. AA is in septic shock with metabolic acidosis and hyperlactatemia. Possible source of infection is community-acquired pneumonia.
  - Resuscitation with a balanced salt solution will be prudent.
  - He should be monitored closely for worsening of hypoxia. After an initial bolus of 500–1000 ml, further fluid boluses should be continued only if he is still fluid responsive (as will be discussed in Chap. 9) and there is continued presence of organ hypoperfusion.
- In case scenario 2, Ms. GA is in hemorrhagic shock possibly due to hemoperitoneum and fracture left femur. With a low GCS, the possibility of traumatic brain injury must be ruled out in this victim of a road traffic accident.
  - 0.9% Saline is possibly the most appropriate resuscitation fluid of choice in this patient with possible associated TBI. Another alternative could be Sterofundin.

**Take-Home Messages**

- Crystalloid formulations used for resuscitation must have tonicity closer to extracellular fluid.
- 0.9% Saline is associated with dilutional, hyperchloremic acidosis with potentially adverse effects on renal perfusion, coagulopathy, GI disturbance and mortality. However, the ill effects of dilutional hyperchloremic acidosis on patient-centred outcomes have not yet been documented unequivocally.
- Overall balanced fluids have an edge over saline especially in larger volume resuscitation with a trend towards improved outcomes in several studies. Rate of fluid, severity of illness, end-organ dysfunction and cost should also be considered while selecting appropriate resuscitation fluid.

- However, 0.9% Saline is the crystalloid of choice in specific circumstances like traumatic brain injury, resuscitation of patients with gastric volume loss and when no other formulation is available (unfortunately not an uncommon scenario in the developing world).
- Hypertonic saline solution has not shown any advantage over isotonic crystalloids in large clinical trials and cannot be recommended for routine use during resuscitation.

## References


1. Chowdhury AH, Cox EF, Francis ST, Lobo DN. A randomized, controlled, double-blind crossover study on the effects of 2-L infusions of 0.9% saline and plasma-yte® 148 on renal blood flow velocity and renal cortical tissue perfusion in healthy volunteers. Ann Surg. 2012;256:18–24.
2. Roquilly A, Loutrel O, Cinotti R, Rosenczweig E, Flet L, Mahe PJ, et al. Balanced versus chloride-rich solutions for fluid resuscitation in brain-injured patients: a randomised double-blind pilot study. Crit Care. 2013;17:R77.
3. Carlesso E, Maiocchi G, Tallarini F, Polli F, Valenza F, Cadringher P, Gattinoni L. The rule regulating pH changes during crystalloid infusion. Intensive Care Med. 2011;37:461–8.
4. O'Malley CM, Frumento RJ, Hardy MA, Benvenisty AI, Brentjens TE, Mercer JS, Bennett-Guerrero E. A randomized, double-blind comparison of lactated Ringer's solution and 0.9% NaCl during renal transplantation. Anesth Analg. 2005;100:1518–24.
5. Khajavi MR, Etezadi F, Moharari RS, Imani F, Meysamie AP, Khashayar P, Najafi A. Effects of normal saline vs. lactated ringer's during renal transplantation. Ren Fail. 2008;30:535–9.
6. Modi MP, Vora KS, Parikh GP, Shah VR. A comparative study of impact of infusion of Ringer's lactate solution versus normal saline on acid-base balance and serum electrolytes during

live related renal transplantation. Saudi J Kidney Dis Transpl. 2012;23:135–7.
7. Yunos NM, Bellomo R, Hegarty C, Story D, Ho L, Bailey M. Association between a chloride-liberal vs chloride-restrictive intravenous fluid administration strategy and kidney injury in critically ill adults. JAMA. 2012;308:1566–72.
8. Raghunathan K, Shaw A, Nathanson B, Stürmer T, Brookhart A, Stefan MS, et al. Association between the choice of IV crystalloid and in-hospital mortality among critically ill adults with sepsis. Crit Care Med. 2014;42:1585–91.
9. Yunos NM, Bellomo R, Glassford N, Sutcliffe H, Lam Q, Bailey M. Chloride-liberal vs. chloride-restrictive intravenous fluid administration and acute kidney injury: an extended analysis. Intensive Care Med. 2015;41:257–64.
10. Young P, Bailey M, Beasley R, Henderson S, Mackle D, McArthur C, et al. Effect of a buffered crystalloid solution vs saline on acute kidney injury among patients in the intensive care unit: the SPLIT randomized clinical trial. JAMA. 2015;314:1701–10.
11. Semler MW, Wanderer JP, Ehrenfeld JM, Stollings JL, Self WH, Siew ED, et al. Balanced crystalloids versus saline in the intensive care unit. The SALT randomized trial. Am J Respir Crit Care Med. 2017;195:1362–72.
12. Semler MW, Self WH, Wanderer JP, Ehrenfeld JM, Wang L, Byrne DW, et al. Balanced crystalloids versus saline in critically ill adults. N Engl J Med. 2018;378:829–39.
13. Self WH, Semler MW, Wanderer JP, Wang L, Byrne DW, Collins SP, et al. Balanced crystalloids versus saline in noncritically ill adults. N Engl J Med. 2018;378:819–28.
14. Zampieri FG, Machado FR, Biondi RS, Freitas FGR, Veiga VC, Figueiredo RC, et al. Effect of intravenous fluid treatment with a balanced solution vs 0.9% saline solution on mortality in critically ill patients: the BaSICS Randomized Clinical Trial. JAMA. 2021;326:818–29.
15. Asfer P, Schortgen F, Boisramé-Helms J, Charpentier J, Guérot E, Megarbane B, et al. Hyperoxia and hypertonic saline in patients with septic shock (HYPERS2S): a two-by-two factorial, multicentre, randomised, clinical trial. Lancet Respir Med. 2017;5:180–90.

# Chapter 6
# Place of Colloids in Resuscitation

## 6.1 Case Scenario

Mr. SG, a 38-year-old male was brought to the emergency department following a road traffic accident. He was managed initially in another hospital where he had received approximately 1.5 litres of 0.9% Saline before transfer and on the way in the ambulance he received another 500 ml of Ringer's lactate. On examination in the ED, he was unconscious with GCS of E1M4V2 and was moving all four limbs. His heart rate was 112/min, blood pressure was 80/40 mmHg. He was having tachypnoea and laboured breathing. Breath sound was significantly diminished in the left hemithorax. Abdomen was distended. His left thigh was swollen with evidence of hematoma. FAST exam was positive for free fluid in the abdomen. The young emergency resident wanted to give some Gelatin infusion before blood products were made available.


S. Ghosh, *Handbook of Intravenous Fluids*,
https://doi.org/10.1007/978-981-19-0500-1_6

### *6.1.1 Is there Any Real Advantage of Colloid Infusion in Acutely Ill Patients?*

Colloids are intravenous fluids containing high molecular weight microscopic substances suspended in crystalloid solutions. Colloids can be classified into two groups: "**Natural**" (albumin solution) and "**Semisynthetic**" (hydroxyethyl starch, gelatin. Dextran solutions). Owing to their high molecular weight, colloid substances only sluggishly cross healthy semi-permeable endothelial barrier and tend to remain in intravascular space for a longer period of time (compared to crystalloids). This way a big advantage of colloid solutions is their significant volume sparing effect. Theoretically volume of colloid required to maintain same intravascular volume is three times lower than crystalloids. But this advantage is lost, albeit to a variable extent, when endothelial glycocalyx is damaged in inflammatory states. Moreover, colloid solutions are expensive and many of them are associated with a number of adverse consequences. In this chapter, we shall discuss the current role of colloid solutions in resuscitation of acutely ill patients.

## 6.2 Albumin

- Albumin is a plasma protein produced exclusively in the liver and participates in a wide range of homeostatic functions in physiological state. Some of the more important roles of albumin are maintaining colloid osmotic pressure of plasma (responsible for 75–80% of colloid osmotic pressure at baseline), maintaining acid–base homeostasis (most important component of anion gap in traditional concept and $A_{TOT}$ in Stewart's concept, as discussed in Chap. 3), as major carrier protein for both endogenous substances (hormones, bilirubin, etc.) or medications (anti-epileptics, digoxin, antibiotics, etc.), as anti-oxidant, anti-inflammatory and anti-apoptotic properties.

- About 9–14 g of albumin is synthesized daily in the liver and a similar amount of albumin is degraded daily in different organs of the body (mostly liver). Dynamics of albumin is shown pictorially in Fig. 6.1.
- Importantly, some of the intravascular albumin move out to the extravascular (interstitial) compartment daily by transcapillary leak and is brought back to the circulation via lymphatics. In inflammatory states, this transcapillary leak increases substantially, overwhelming the capacity of lymphatics, ultimately resulting in hypoalbuminemia.
- Hypoalbuminemia is further complicated by reduced hepatic production of albumin in acutely ill patients.

• Interestingly, there is a large body of literature available showing an association between hypoalbuminemia and mortality in acutely ill patients [1].

• Commercially albumin is produced by fractionation of human plasma, which is heat-treated further to reduce transmission of blood-borne pathogens. It is available as

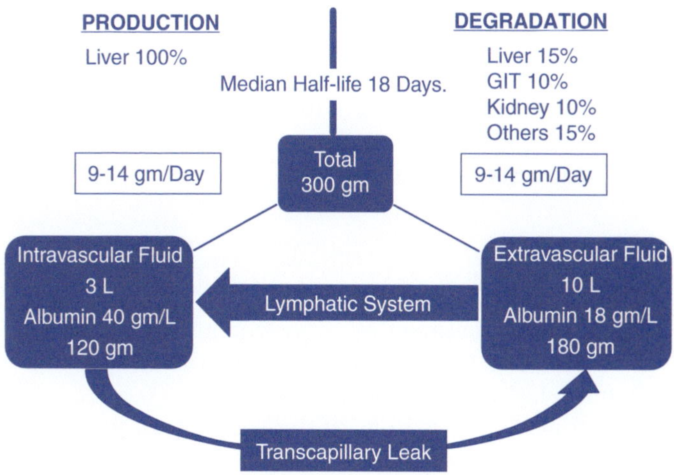


FIGURE 6.1 Albumin dynamics in physiological state

both hypo- (iso-osmotic) 4 or 5% Solution and hyperoncotic 20 or 25% solution. It is expensive, may not be made available widely and has the potential for allergic reactions.

- Role of albumin infusion is well established in conditions like spontaneous bacterial peritonitis, hepatorenal syndrome, during large-volume paracentesis in patients with chronic liver disease or during plasma exchange. Albumin also have potential role during de-resuscitation and will be discussed further in Chap. 10. There may be some role of albumin in the management of burn victims in the later stage and will be discussed in Chap. 14.

- In subsequent paragraphs, we shall discuss "**5 Points to Remember**" for Albumin resuscitation in acutely Ill patients.

1. Overall, it is safe to use albumin infusion in critically ill patients.
   - This obvious fact was challenged by a Cochrane review published in 1998 [2]. In a meta-analysis of 30 small, highly heterogenous and poorly performed RCTs, the review erroneously concluded that infusion of albumin is associated with an overall 6% increase in mortality [2].
   - However, the results of that meta-analysis were comprehensively nullified by landmark "**SAFE**" study (discussed in Box 6.1) [3].

**Box 6.1 "SAFE" Study** [3]

- **Research Question:** Does resuscitation with albumin differs from saline resuscitation in terms of all-cause mortality of ICU patients at 28 days?
- **Setting:** 16 ICUs from Australia and New Zealand participated in the trial.

- **Patient:** 6997 Patients who required volume resuscitation within 28 days of ICU admission were randomized to one of the two following groups.
- **Intervention:** 4% Albumin for resuscitation.
- **Control:** 0.9% Saline for resuscitation.
- **Outcome:** Albumin group received less fluid in the first 4 days. But the ratio of Saline to Albumin 1:1.4 (not 1:3 as expected theoretically).
  - Albumin resuscitation does not increase 28-days mortality compared to 0.9% Saline (20.9% versus 21.1%) [Primary Outcome].
  - No difference in secondary outcome measures like ICU or hospital length of stay, mechanical ventilation days or days on renal replacement therapy between two groups.
  - In subgroup analysis, patients with sepsis had a trend towards better outcome with Albumin resuscitation. In contrast, albumin resuscitation in trauma patients (especially with traumatic brain injury) was associated with more death.

2. Patients with sepsis may be benefited by albumin infusion. This conclusion could be drawn from a follow-up study of sepsis patients from SAFE cohort that showed better-adjusted mortality at 28 days in albumin group [4]. However, this conclusion needs to be balanced against high cost and scarce availability of albumin.
3. It is not safe to use albumin as resuscitation fluid in patients with traumatic brain injury, demonstrated clearly in "**SAFE-TBI**" Study (Box 6.2) [5]. Possible explanation for this increase in mortality with albumin could be because of an increase in vasogenic or cytotoxic oedema in patients with damaged blood–brain barrier. This explanation is valid for other colloids too.

**Box 6.2 "SAFE-TBI" Study** [5]

- **Research Question:** Is there any difference between albumin and saline resuscitation on all-cause mortality and neurological outcome in patients with TBI?
- **Methods:** 460 Patients with TBI from SAFE study cohort were followed up for 24 months and the mortality and neurological outcome were recorded at the end of observation period.
  - 231 patients were in the 4% Albumin group and 229 patients in the 0.9% Saline group.
- **Outcome:** Patients in albumin group had higher mortality at 24 months compared to 0.9% Saline (33.2% vs 20.4%) and the result remains the same even after adjustment for baseline covariates.
  - The effect was more pronounced in patients with severe TBI (GCS 8 or below at baseline).
  - Patients in albumin group had significantly worse Glasgow outcome score at 24 months. Again, the effect was more pronounced in patients with severe TBI.

4. In an observational study, rapid infusion of hyperoncotic albumin was shown to increase intravascular volume by two times the infusion volume in patients with septic shock [6]. The volume expansion effect reached its peak at 30 minute and persisted even at 4 hours.
   - Similar volume expansion effect of 20% Albumin could be seen in "**SWIPE**" Study (Box 6.3) [7].
   - Based on these data hyperoncotic albumin infusion may be considered in selected patients of septic shock, where the need for crystalloid infusion is judged to be too high (with an ultimate aim to reduce the cumulative fluid balance).

**Box 6.3 "SWIPE" Study** [7]

- **Research Question:** Can resuscitation with 20% Albumin compared to 4–5% Albumin decrease the volume of resuscitation fluid and be associated with less cumulative fluid volume?
- **Setting:** 3 ICUs from Australia and UK. New.
- **Patient:** 321 Patients requiring fluid bolus within 48-hour of ICU admission.
- **Intervention:** 20% Albumin for volume expansion.
- **Control:** 4% (in Australia) or 5% (in UK) Albumin for volume expansion.
- **Outcome:** Intravascular volume expansion effect of 20% Albumin was >2-times higher compared to 4 or 5% Albumin (100 ml ~275 ml).
  - Cumulative volume of resuscitation fluid at 48-hour was significantly lower in the 20% albumin group compared to the 4 or 5% albumin group (median difference 600 ml).
  - 20% albumin group had lower overall cumulative fluid balance at 48-hour.
  - There was no difference in duration of mechanical ventilation and need for renal replacement therapy between two groups.
  - There was a small but significant difference in the proportion of patients discharged alive from ICU between two groups favouring 20% albumin group (97.4% versus 91.1%).
- **Limitation:** Apart from small size the study was limited by disproportionate representation of elective surgery patients (about 80%) and only small percentage of patients with sepsis (about 17%).

5. In patients with septic shock, the role of albumin may go beyond just volume expansion.
   - In a post-hoc analysis of "**ALBIOS**" study, albumin infusion started within 24 hours of sepsis onset with a target to maintain serum albumin level above 3 g/L, was found to reduce mortality in subgroup of patients with septic shock [8]. This beneficial effect observed could probably be attributed to physiological effects of albumin, other than just maintaining osmolality, including ant-oxidant or anti-inflammatory effects [9].
   - In a small study on patients with septic shock, 20% Albumin infusion was found to improve endothelial activity (assessed by endothelial response to acetylcholine) by twofold compared to infusion of 0.9% saline [10].

## 6.3 Hydroxyethyl Starch (HES)

- HES solutions are semisynthetic colloids produced by hydroxyethyl substitution of amylopectin molecules present in starches. Hydroxyethyl substitution protects amylopectin molecules from degradation by amylases present in plasma, thus prolonging their osmotic effect.
- Amylopectin molecules are obtained from natural sources like sorghum, maize or potatoes. Effects (and adverse effects) of HES depend on the following chemical properties of the solution and are displayed in the commercially available preparation as numbers:
  - Concentration of HES in the solution (e.g. 6%, 10%)
  - Median molecular weight of the HES molecule (e.g. 130, 200 Kilo Dalton)
  - Degree of molecular substitution (e.g. tetrastarch, pentastarch)
  - Ratio of hydroxyethyl substitution at C2 and C6 carbon atoms of glucose subunit (C2/C6 ratio)
  - Carrier fluid (like 0.9% NaCl, e.g. Voluven or balanced fluid, e.g. Volulyte)

- ***Higher concentration and higher molecular weight of HES are associated with greater osmotic effect but at the same time, these properties are also associated with changes in viscoelastic measurements and fibrinolysis, producing increased coagulopathy.***
- ***Higher degree of substitution and higher C2/C6 ratio offer better protection against amylases of blood at a cost of increased accumulation in reticuloendothelial tissues like skin, liver, kidneys.***
- Types of carrier fluid can have a significant impact on acid–base balance.
- ***Number of adverse effects are associated with the use of HES including worsening of renal functions, coagulopathy, itching (may last for years) and allergic reactions.***
- In more recent years HES solutions have fallen out of favour because worsening organ functions and possible increase in mortality seen with its use in well-conducted randomized control trials, especially in septic shock. Table 6.1 summarizes the findings of three large randomized trials of HES versus crystalloids done on patients with sepsis.
- ***Based on these evidences, HES solutions should not be used in patients with septic shock.***

- HES solutions are still being used in perioperative settings, despite insufficient data supporting its use in this setting [14]. ***With no benefit observed in patient-centric outcomes in large RCTs, possible adverse effects associated with the use of HES and substantial increase in cost (compared to crystalloids), use of HES should be discouraged even in perioperative setting.***
- ***HES should not be used in patients with trauma or with any form of brain injury.*** In a retrospective review of 2225 trauma patients, resuscitation with 6% Hetastarch was associated with an increased incidence of acute kidney injury and increased mortality [15].

TABLE 6.1 Randomized trials comparing HES solutions versus crystalloids in septic shock resuscitation

| | **VISEP study** [11] | **6-S study** [12] | **CHEST study** [13] |
|---|---|---|---|
| Setting | 18-German ICUs | 26-Scandinavian ICUs | 32-ICUs ANZ. |
| No of patients | 537 | 798 | 6651 |
| Patient group | Severe sepsis or septic shock. | Severe sepsis | All ICU patients requiring resuscitation. |
| Intervention | HES 200/0.5 in balanced salt solution. | HES 130/0.42 in ringer acetate | 6% HES (130/0.4) in saline. |
| Control | Ringer's lactate. | Ringer acetate. | 0.9% saline. |
| Primary outcome | No difference in 28-day mortality | HES—Higher death or dialysis dependent at Day 90 | No difference in mortality at Day 90. |
| Secondary outcome | Trend towards increased 90-day mortality in HES. HES—Increased AKI and need for RRT. | No difference in mortality at Day 28. HES—increased need for RRT, worse renal SOFA. | HES—Increased renal and hepatic dysfunction. Saline—Increased cardiovascular dysfunction. |

## 6.4 Gelatins

- Gelatins are colloid solutions containing semisynthetic polypeptides derived from bovine collagen molecules with relatively smaller particle sizes compared to other synthetic colloids (average molecular weight ~ 35,000 Dalton).
- Because of its lower molecular weight colloid osmotic effect of gelatins lasts for a shorter period of time compared to other colloids.
- Two types of gelatin products are available commercially—**Urea cross-linked or polygeline (Haemacel)** or **Succinylated Gelatins (Gelofusine)**.
- There is no well-performed randomized trial data available comparing resuscitation with gelatin solutions versus crystalloids. However, a systematic review of limited studies does not find any advantage of gelatin administration over crystalloids [16].
- Moreover, the use of gelatin is found to be associated with an increase in anaphylaxis and a trend towards increase in bleeding risk, acute kidney injury and mortality [17].
- ***In the absence of any substantial beneficial effect against crystalloids, potential for systemic adverse effects and substantial cost involved with its use, gelatin cannot be recommended as a resuscitation fluid in any acute care setting.***

## 6.5 Dextrans

- Dextrans are hardly being used as volume expander. They are a mixture of glucose polymers of variable sizes, derived from bacteria *Leuconostoc mesenteroides*.
  - Commercially available formulations are 10% Dextran-40 and 6% Dextran-70.
- Based on their sizes dextrans can be classified as either Dextran-40 (average molecular weight 40 Kilo Dalton) or Dextran-70 (average molecular weight 70 Kilo Dalton).

- The duration of colloid osmotic effect depends on size of the particle, with higher molecular weight staying in the intravascular compartment for a longer period of time (average duration Dextran-40 ~ 5 hours and Dextran-70 ~ 6–8 Hours).
- Dextrans are almost exclusively excreted renally with only a small fraction getting eliminated via the gastrointestinal tract.
- A systematic review of limited evidence available comparing Dextrans with crystalloids, no difference could be found in patient-centric clinical outcomes between them in acutely ill patients [16].
- Moreover, Dextrans are associated with renal failure, allergic reactions and coagulopathy.
- ***With little evidence to show any advantage, potential for a number of adverse effects and increased cost, Dextrans should not be used for volume resuscitation***.
  - However, Dextrans are being used in vascular surgery for its unique rheologic properties, decreasing blood viscosity potentially improving microvascular flow, especially after grafting.

## 6.6 Case Scenario (Continued)

- Mr. SG is a victim of road traffic accident with polytrauma and possible traumatic brain injury.
  - He should be resuscitated with crystalloids following principles of "Damage Control Resuscitation" as discussed further in Chap. 12.
  - Massive transfusion protocol should be initiated.
  - Colloids should be strictly avoided, as they are clearly shown to be unsafe for resuscitation of trauma victims especially in patients with TBI.

**Take-Home Messages**

- Colloids have a limited role as resuscitation fluid.
- Volume sparing effect of colloids shown in non-critically ill patients and in healthy volunteers is not replicated to that extent in acutely ill patients.
- Overall, albumin is safe as resuscitation fluid except in patients with trauma in general and brain injury in particular. The adverse consequences of albumin observed in TBI victims can be extrapolated to other patients with cerebral oedema and raised intracranial pressure.
- Hyperoncotic albumin may have some role in limiting resuscitation fluid volume. However, further studies are required to firmly establish this point.
- Use of semisynthetic colloids should be avoided during resuscitation given their potential adverse effects and additional cost without any advantage seen in studies.

## References

1. Vincent JL, Dubois MJ, Navickis RJ, Wilkes MM. Hypoalbuminemia in acute illness: is there a rationale for intervention? A meta-analysis of cohort studies and controlled trials. Ann Surg. 2003;237:319–34.
2. Cochrane Injuries Group Albumin Reviewers. Human albumin administration in critically ill patients: systematic review of randomised controlled trials. BMJ. 1998;317:235–40.
3. Finfer S, Bellomo R, Boyce N, French J, Myburgh J, Norton R, SAFE Study Investigators. A comparison of albumin and saline for fluid resuscitation in the intensive care unit. N Engl J Med. 2004;350:2247–56.

4. Finfer S, McEvoy S, Bellomo R, McArthur C, Myburgh J, Norton R. Impact of albumin compared to saline on organ function and mortality of patients with severe sepsis. Intensive Care Med. 2011;37:86–96.
5. Myburgh J, Cooper DJ, Finfer S, Bellomo R, Norton R, Bishop N, Kai Lo S, Vallance S. Saline or albumin for fluid resuscitation in patients with traumatic brain injury. N Engl J Med. 2007;357:874–84.
6. Margarson MP, Soni NC. Changes in serum albumin concentration and volume expanding effects following a bolus of albumin 20% in septic patients. Br J Anaesth. 2004;92:821–6.
7. Mårtensson J, Bihari S, Bannard-Smith J, Glassford NJ, Lloyd-Donald P, Cioccari L, et al. Small volume resuscitation with 20% albumin in intensive care: physiological effects: the SWIPE randomised clinical trial. Intensive Care Med. 2018;44:1797–806.
8. Caironi P, Tognoni G, Masson S, Fumagalli R, Pesenti A, Romero M, et al. Albumin replacement in patients with severe sepsis or septic shock. N Engl J Med. 2014;370:1412–21.
9. Caironi P. POINT: should intravenous albumin be used for volume resuscitation in severe sepsis/septic shock? Yes Chest. 2016;149:1365–7.
10. Hariri G, Joffre J, Deryckere S, Bigé N, Dumas G, Baudel JL, et al. Albumin infusion improves endothelial function in septic shock patients: a pilot study. Intensive Care Med. 2018;44:669–71.
11. Brunkhorst FM, Engel C, Bloos F, Meier-Hellmann A, Ragaller M, Weiler N, et al. Intensive insulin therapy and pentastarch resuscitation in severe sepsis. N Engl J Med. 2008;358:125–39.
12. Perner A, Haase N, Guttormsen AB, Tenhunen J, Klemenzson G, Åneman A, et al. Hydroxyethyl starch 130/0.42 versus Ringer's acetate in severe sepsis. N Engl J Med. 2012;367:124–34.
13. Myburgh JA, Finfer S, Bellomo R, Billot L, Cass A, Gattas D, et al. Hydroxyethyl starch or saline for fluid resuscitation in intensive care. N Engl J Med. 2012;367:1901–11.
14. Raiman M, Mitchell CG, Biccard BM, Rodseth RN. Comparison of hydroxyethyl starch colloids with crystalloids for surgical patients: a systematic review and meta-analysis. Eur J Anaesthesiol. 2016;33:42–8.
15. Lissauer ME, Chi A, Kramer ME, Scalea TM, Johnson SB. Association of 6% Hetastarch resuscitation with adverse outcomes in critically ill trauma patients. Am J Surg. 2011;202:53–8.

16. Lewis SR, Pritchard MW, Evans DJW, Butler AR, Alderson P, Smith AF, Roberts I. Colloids versus crystalloids for fluid resuscitation in critically ill people. Cochrane Database Syst Rev. 2018;8:CD000567.
17. Moeller C, Fleischmann C, Thomas-Rueddel D, Vlasakov V, Rochwerg B, Theurer P, Gattinoni L, Reinhart K, Hartog CS. How safe is gelatin? A systematic review and meta-analysis of gelatin-containing plasma expanders vs crystalloids and albumin. J Crit Care. 2016;35:75–83.

# Chapter 7
# Maintenance Fluid

## 7.1 Case Scenario 1

Mr. AB, a 65-year-old previously hypertensive male got admitted to the ICU with large left middle cerebral artery territory infarct. He weighed about 75 kg. His GCS is E2M5V1 with aphasia and right hemiplegia. Clinically he looks euvolemic. His heart rate is 108 per minute with atrial fibrillation as underlying rhythm and blood pressure is 156/100 mmHg. Rest of the systemic examination is unremarkable. He is started on 20% Mannitol boluses by the neurology team. Considering the potentially compromised airway, the intensive care team decides to keep him nil by mouth till further order.

## 7.2 Case Scenario 2

Ms. PG, a 28-year-old previously healthy woman was admitted to the high dependency unit with pain upper abdomen and vomiting of 1-day duration. Her body weight is 50 kg. She was diagnosed with acute cholecystitis and planned to be managed medically with intravenous ceftriaxone, metronidazole, titrated dose of fentanyl infusion and maintenance intravenous fluid. Considering her poor oral intake for the past


S. Ghosh, *Handbook of Intravenous Fluids*,
https://doi.org/10.1007/978-981-19-0500-1_7

several hours, she was given an intravenous bolus of 1000 ml Lactated Ringer's solution in the Emergency Department. Currently, she looks euvolemic with normal peripheral perfusion. Her initial laboratory investigations reveal normal values of serum electrolytes.

### *7.2.1 How do We Plan Maintenance Fluid Prescription in Different Clinical Scenarios?*

Maintenance intravenous fluids are prescribed for fulfilling fluid and electrolytes requirements of an individual, when he or she is unable to take anything by mouth or enterally. Recent research showed that maintenance fluids account for almost a fourth of daily fluid volume received by an intensive care unit patient and contribute significantly to cumulative fluid balance [1]. Prescription of maintenance fluid must be balanced carefully against the potential harm of producing positive cumulative fluid balance. The prescription should consider appropriate indication, volume and electrolyte (especially sodium and potassium) requirements of the patient and glucose supplement (to counter starvation ketoacidosis) and tonicity of the fluid prescribed. Initial prescription should be modified periodically based on clinical assessment of the patient, electrolyte concentration of serum and further need for maintenance fluid prescription altogether. In this chapter, we shall be discussing about indications for maintenance fluids, type and volume of fluid to be prescribed and what to monitor during ongoing maintenance fluid treatment.

## 7.3 Who Needs Maintenance Fluid?

- Maintenance fluid prescription should be strictly limited to patients who cannot take sufficient volume of fluid orally or by enteral route because of profound nausea or vomiting or when patients are being kept nil by mouth for some medical reason.

- Patients on maintenance fluids must be assessed periodically for possibility of recommencing oral or enteral feeding (fluid intake).
- Some typical indications of maintenance fluid prescription are perioperative scenario (often for a more than necessary period), patients with acute abdomen, patients with potential airway compromise, etc.

## 7.4 Which Fluid?

- Traditionally maintenance fluids prescribed were hypotonic fluids with low sodium and chloride with an appropriate amount of potassium and glucose. These recommendations were based on physiological experiments by Holiday and Segar [2].
- More recently, these traditional concepts have been challenged because of the concern for hyponatremia resulting from low sodium hypotonic fluid prescription.
- Some concerns have also been raised about cerebral oedema and seizure associated with hyponatremia and possible persistent neurological damage resulting from the same [3]. Later concern was raised mostly in paediatric patient population.
  - In a systematic review and meta-analysis of 10 randomized control trials including total of 823 patients, authors evaluated the incidence of hyponatremia in children on either isotonic or hypotonic maintenance fluid [4]. *Hypotonic fluid prescription was associated with higher incidences of both mild (<135 mEq/L) and moderate (<130 mEq/L) hyponatremia. However, there was no difference in terms of cerebral oedema and neurological adverse effects between these two groups* [4].
  - Three more recent RCTs [5–7] evaluated the effects of isotonic or moderately hypotonic maintenance fluids on hyponatremia and other electrolytes abnormalities and are summarized in Table 7.1.

TABLE 7.1 Recent RCTs comparing isotonic versus moderately hypotonic maintenance intravenous fluids in paediatric age group

| | **McNab et al. [5]** | **Friedman et al. [6]** | **Lehtiranta et al. [7]** |
|---|---|---|---|
| Setting | Single centre. Australia | Single centre. USA | Single centre. Finland |
| No of patients | 690 | 110 | 614 |
| Patient group | 3 months to 18 years Requiring intravenous maintenance fluid >6 h | 1 month to 18 years Requiring intravenous maintenance fluid >48 h | 6 months to 12 years Requiring intravenous maintenance fluid. |
| Intervention | Plasmalyte 148 plus 5% Dextrose | 0.9% Saline plus 5% Dextrose | Plasmalyte 148 plus 5% Dextrose |
| Control | 0.45% Saline plus 5% Dextrose | 0.45% Saline plus 5% Dextrose | Commercial solution containing 80 mmol/L Na, 20 mmol/L K plus 5% Dextrose |
| Primary outcome | Lower hyponatremia (Na <135 mmol/L) incidence in isotonic group. 4% versus 11%. | No difference in mean sodium level at 48 h. 139.9 mmol/L in isotonic vs. 139.6 mmol/L in hypotonic. | Higher clinically significant electrolyte disorders (Na <132 mmol/L or >148 mmol/L or K <3.5 mmol/L) isotonic group. 20% vs. 2.9% |

Table 7.1 (continued)

| | **McNab et al.** [5] | **Friedman et al.** [6] | **Lehtiranta et al.** [7] |
|---|---|---|---|
| Secondary outcome | No difference in hypernatremia. Numerically higher incidence of seizure in hypotonic group. No difference in cerebral edema. More adverse events in isotonic group including one instance of clinical fluid overload. | No difference in mean sodium level at 24-h. No difference in overall hyponatremia and hypernatremia. No difference in change of weight at 24 h and at 48 h. Modestly higher change in mean sodium value from baseline in hypotonic group. | Higher hypokalaemia in isotonic group.19% vs. 2.9% Higher hypernatremia in isotonic group.1.3% vs. 0% No difference in clinically significant hyponatremia. Greater weight gain associated with isotonic fluid. No difference in neurological complications. |

- Potential risk of hyponatremia (mostly mild, asymptomatic) with hypotonic fluid infusion must be balanced against the risk of volume overload resulting from isotonic sodium-rich fluid [8] and risk of hypokalaemia with prescription of potassium poor commercially available isotonic maintenance solutions.
  - Another pertinent question is whether results from paediatric studies be extrapolated to adult population.
  - In the lone RCT comparing isotonic and hypotonic maintenance fluid in adults (Box 7.1 below), no differ-

ence was observed in significant hyponatremia incidence between groups; but significantly higher incidence clinical fluid overload was observed in isotonic fluid group resulting in premature discontinuation of the study [9].

**Box 7.1 "Topmast" study** [9]

- **Research Question**: Does infusion of maintenance fluid containing 154 mmol/L sodium produces more fluid retention compared to a solution containing 54 mmol/L sodium following major surgery.
- **Setting:** Single centre from Belgium.
- **Patient:** 70 Patients undergoing major thoracic surgery. Patients with glomerular filtration rate <60 ml/kg/1.73 $m^2$) or on diuretics or any form of nutrition were excluded from the study.
- **Intervention:** isotonic maintenance fluid: Received 0.9% Saline with 5% Dextrose (Na-154 Group).
- **Control:** Hypotonic maintenance fluid: Received Glucion 5% containing 54 mmol/L Sodium (Na-54 Group).
- **Outcome:** At 72 h, Na-154 group had mean of 1369 mL more positive balance compared to Na-54 group. Non-study fluid volume in both groups was similar.
  - 11.8% of patients in Na-54 groups had mild hyponatremia (Na <135 mmol/L) compared to none in Na-154 group.
  - But incidences of more significant hyponatremia (Na <130 mmol/L) were not different between groups.
  - There was more hyperchloremia (Cl > 109 mmol/L) in Na-154 group.
  - Six patients in Na-154 group (compared to one patient in Na-54 group) developed clinical or radiographic fluid overload forcing investigators to discontinue the study.

- Even in paediatric patients, isotonic fluids tend to produce more volume overload compared to moderately hypotonic fluids as documented clearly in the study by Lehtiranta and colleagues. Deleterious effects of positive cumulative fluid balance and volume overload on clinical outcomes of patients are now well established [10, 11].
- Underlying clinical conditions also should be considered while prescribing maintenance intravenous fluid. For example, prescription of hypotonic fluid can potentially worsen cerebral edema in a patient with brain injury or sodium-rich fluids can worsen heart failure in a patient with left ventricular dysfunction.
- Table 7.2 below summarizes composition of different commercially available and commonly prescribed maintenance intravenous fluids. Notably, Plasmalyte 148 with 5% Dextrose and Glucion-5% (both commercially manufactured by Baxter healthcare) are not available in the Indian market.

## 7.5 How Much Fluid?

- Prescription of maintenance intravenous fluid should consider three different but inter-related aspects: daily maintenance volume, daily requirements of electrolytes especially sodium and potassium and daily glucose need to counter starvation ketoacidosis [12].
- An approach to calculating initial maintenance intravenous fluid is given below (adapted from the United Kingdom, National Health Services Guidelines):
  - Daily maintenance volume: 25–30 ml/kg body weight per day
  - Sodium: 1–2 mmol/kg/day
  - Potassium: 1 mmol/kg/day
  - Chloride: 1–2 mmol/kg/day
  - Glucose: 50 to 100 g per day

TABLE 7.2 Composition of commonly prescribed maintenance intravenous fluids

| | **5% Dextrose +0.9% saline** | **5% Dextrose + plasmalyte-148** | **5% Dextrose +0.45% saline** | **Isolyte-M** | **Isolyte-P** | **Glucion-5%** |
|---|---|---|---|---|---|---|
| Sodium (mmol/L) | 154 | 140 | 77 | 40 | 25 | 54 |
| Potassium (mmol/L) | – | 5 | – | 35 | 20 | 26 |
| Chloride (mmol/L) | 154 | 98 | 77 | 38 | 22 | 55 |
| Phosphate (mmol/L) | – | – | – | 15 | 3 | 6.2 |
| Magnesium (mmol/L) | – | 1.5 | – | – | 3 | 2.6 |
| Lactate (mmol/L) | | – | | | | 25 |
| Acetate (mmol/L) | – | 27 | – | 20 | 23 | |
| Gluconate (mmol/L) | – | 23 | | | | |
| Glucose (gm/L) | 50 | 50 | 50 | 50 | 50 | 50 |

- In obese patients, fluid prescription should be based on ideal body weight. Total volume of maintenance fluid normally should not exceed 3 litres per day [12].
- In children, volume of fluid is calculated from Holiday and Segar formula (as depicted below) [2]:
  - For first 10 Kg weight: 100 ml/kg/day
  - For 10–20 Kg weight: Additional 50 ml/kg/day
  - For weight above 20 Kg: Additional 20 ml/kg/day
- Initial volume of prescribed fluid should be lower in patients with congestive heart failure, renal dysfunction and in malnourished patients—may be approximately 20–30 ml/kg/day [12].

## 7.6 Monitoring

- Initial rate of fluid infusion should be adjusted periodically based on the patient's ongoing clinical status. Following parameters should be monitored to adjust maintenance fluid dose.
  - Tissue perfusion including sensorium, peripheral perfusion and urine output (but none of them in isolation)
  - Ongoing fluid loss. Examples, diarrhoea, vomiting, haemorrhage, increased insensible loss due to high fever or tachypnoea
  - Daily fluid balance or balance between total fluid intake (including resuscitation, maintenance, replacement, fluids used as drug diluent and flushing vascular catheter and nutritional fluid) minus total output (including urine output, output from different drains, ultrafiltration and fluids removed by paracentesis)
  - Daily weight of the patient (if possible)
  - Serum electrolytes particularly serum sodium and potassium. Sometimes magnesium, calcium and phosphate
  - Arterial blood gases for base excess, metabolic acidosis or alkalosis

## 7.7 Case Scenario (Continued)

- Mr. AB is at a high risk of hyponatremia and worsening cerebral oedema with hypotonic fluid prescription and should receive only isotonic maintenance fluid.
  - The best commercially available fluid for him will be 5% Dextrose with 0.9% Saline.
  - Initial fluid prescription should consist of approximately 2250 ml of fluid per day at a rate of /hour.
  - He is also at a higher risk of hypokalaemia because of ongoing treatment with mannitol and potassium should be added to the solution.
  - He should be monitored carefully for electrolytes especially sodium and potassium and for additional fluid loss because of osmotic diuresis.
- As discussed in the text above, most appropriate maintenance fluid for Ms. PG will be a moderately hypotonic fluid.
  - She will require approximately 1500 ml of volume with 100 mmol sodium and 50 mmol potassium per day.
  - In addition, she will require 100 gm of glucose in her prescription.
  - 1500 ml of 0.45% Saline with 5% Dextrose **PLUS** 10 ml of 15% Potassium chloride solution (containing 20 mEq Potassium/10 ml) added to each 500 ml of solution, over 24 h should be able to fulfil these requirements.
  - She should be monitored for urine output, ongoing requirement of replacement fluid and electrolyte abnormalities.

**Take-Home Messages**
- Maintenance fluids contribute significantly to positive cumulative fluid balance and great amount of caution should be applied while prescribing maintenance intravenous fluid including right indication,

right volume and right choice of fluid. Patients should be switched to oral or enteral feeding and maintenance fluid should be discontinued at the earliest instance.

- In adult patients, hypotonic fluid with low sodium with adequate amount of glucose and potassium should suffice for maintenance fluid needs. This prescription should be able to limit cumulative fluid balance.
- In children, prescription of maintenance intravenous fluid should balance between the risk of hyponatremia (mostly mild and asymptomatic) versus potential for volume overload, hypernatremia and hypokalaemia. Even in children, perhaps, prescription of moderately hypotonic fluid should be preferred. However, children on maintenance infusion should be monitored more carefully with serial assessment of weight, cumulative fluid balance and electrolytes.
- In patients at a higher risk of cerebral edema maintenance fluid prescribed should be isotonic.
- Prescription of fluid volume and electrolytes should be based on ideal body weight. Patients at a higher risk of volume overload should be prescribed lower volume.
- Prescription of maintenance fluid must also take into account other concomitant sources of fluids and electrolytes the patient is receiving—including enteral and parenteral nutrition, fluids administered as drug diluents and fluids used to flush intravascular lines.
- Patients must be frequently monitored while on maintenance fluid infusion for peripheral perfusion, ongoing volume loss and electrolytes especially serum sodium and potassium levels.

## References


1. Van Regenmortel N, Verbrugghe W, Roelant E, Van den Wyngaert T, Jorens PG. Maintenance fluid therapy and fluid creep impose more significant fluid, sodium, and chloride burdens than resuscitation fluids in critically ill patients: a retrospective study in a tertiary mixed ICU population. Intensive Care Med. 2018;44:409–17.
2. Holliday MA, Segar WE. The maintenance need for water in parenteral fluid therapy. Pediatrics. 1957;19:823–32.
3. Hughes PD, McNicol D, Mutton PM, Flynn GJ, Tuck R, Yorke P. Postoperative hyponatraemic encephalopathy: water intoxication. Intravenous fluids for seriously ill children: time to reconsider. Lancet. 2003;362:1320–3.
4. Foster BA, Tom D, Hill V. Hypotonic versus isotonic fluids in hospitalized children: a systematic review and meta-analysis. J Pediatr. 2014;165:163–9.
5. McNab S, Duke T, South M, Babl FE, Lee KJ, Arnup SJ, et al. 140 mmol/L of sodium versus 77 mmol/L of sodium in maintenance intravenous fluid therapy for children in hospital (PIMS): a randomised controlled double-blind trial. Lancet. 2015;385:1190–7.
6. Friedman JN, Beck CE, DeGroot J, Geary DF, Sklansky DJ, Freedman SB. Comparison of isotonic and hypotonic intravenous maintenance fluids: a randomized clinical trial. JAMA Pediatr. 2015;169:445–51.
7. Lehtiranta S, Honkila M, Kallio M, Paalanne N, Peltoniemi O, Pokka T, Renko M, Tapiainen T. Risk of electrolyte disorders in acutely ill children receiving commercially available plasmalike isotonic fluids: a randomized clinical trial. JAMA Pediatr. 2021;175:28–35.
8. Van Regenmortel N, Jorens PG. Effect of isotonic vs hypotonic maintenance fluid therapy on urine output, fluid balance, and electrolyte homeostasis: a crossover study in fasting adult volunteers. Reply from the authors. Br J Anaesth. 2017;119:1065–7.
9. Van Regenmortel N, Hendrickx S, Roelant E, Baar I, Dams K, Van Vlimmeren K, et al. 154 compared to 54 mmol per liter of sodium in intravenous maintenance fluid therapy for adult patients undergoing major thoracic surgery (TOPMAST): a single-center randomized controlled double-blind trial. Intensive Care Med. 2019;45:1422–32.

10. Boyd JH, Forbes J, Nakada TA, Walley KR, Russell JA. Fluid resuscitation in septic shock: a positive fluid balance and elevated central venous pressure are associated with increased mortality. Crit Care Med. 2011;39:259–65.
11. Silversides JA, Fitzgerald E, Manickavasagam US, Lapinsky SE, Nisenbaum R, Hemmings N, et al. Role of active deresuscitation after resuscitation (RADAR) investigators. Deresuscitation of patients with iatrogenic fluid overload is associated with reduced mortality in critical illness. Crit Care Med. 2018;46:1600–7.
12. Padhi S, Bullock I, Li L, Stroud M. Intravenous fluid therapy for adults in hospital: summary of NICE guidance. BMJ. 2013;347:f7073.

# Chapter 8
# Vasopressors in Resuscitation

## 8.1 Case Vignette

Mr. VG, a 74-year-old male with past history of diabetes mellitus, hypertension and obstructive sleep apnoea on domiciliary bipap is admitted to the ICU with increasing breathlessness and history suggestive of lower respiratory tract infection, possibly pneumonia. On examination, he is drowsy but arousable, following simple commands with cold peripheries. His capillary refill time is prolonged (>6 seconds), heart rate 124/min regular, blood pressure 84/36 mmHg. ABG shows significant hypoxemia with combined metabolic and respiratory acidosis plus high lactate (6 mmol/L). He has received 500 ml of 0.9% Saline in the ED and another 500 ml of Ringer's lactate is on flow.

### *8.1.1 Vasopressors - Is there Any Right Timing or Right Agent or Right Target?*

Vasopressors are an integral part of resuscitation, used very often along with fluid boluses and infusions. In this chapter, we shall be discussing the role of vasopressors during



S. Ghosh, *Handbook of Intravenous Fluids*,
https://doi.org/10.1007/978-981-19-0500-1_8

resuscitation, appropriate timing of vasopressor initiation, vasopressors commonly used in clinical practice and what should be the target level of blood pressure. Large body of evidence is now available on vasopressor use in patients with septic shock. However, for other situations, the available evidence is still limited.

## 8.2 When to Start

- Surviving sepsis guideline recommends starting vasopressors early (within 1-h) in patients with septic shock, if he or she does not achieve hemodynamic resuscitation goal after the initial fluid bolus [1]. European consensus guideline also recommends starting vasopressors early, even before completion of full fluid resuscitation [2]. However, despite these recommendations, acute care physicians are still more comfortable starting vasopressor infusion only when hemodynamic parameters are still not improving after infusion of large volume of fluid.
- In subsequent paragraphs, we shall be discussing **"5-Good Reasons"** why vasopressor infusion should not be delayed especially in patients with septic shock.
- 1. Prolonged hypotension is harmful and should be avoided. One retrospective study had shown that terminal cardiovascular collapse occurs in systolic, mean and diastolic blood pressures of 47, 35 and 29 mmHg, respectively [3].

    - In a study of patients with post-partum haemorrhage, troponin values were shown to rise at a systolic pressure below 80 mmHg or diastolic pressure below 50 mmHg [4].
    - In a retrospective analysis of 213 patients with septic shock, Bai and colleagues had observed a 5.3% increase in mortality for every 1-h delay in norepinephrine initiation during the first 6 h of resuscitation [5]. In the same study, early initiation (within 2-h) of norepinephrine lowered the duration of hypotension, achieved faster lactate clearance and

was associated with 10% less cumulative fluid balance in first 24 h, lower cumulative 24-h dose of norepinephrine and lower 28-day mortality [5].
- In single-centre CENSER randomized study, early initiation of low-dose norepinephrine infusion along with standard resuscitation measures was shown to achieve faster shock reversal (mean arterial pressure > 65 PLUS adequate tissue perfusion characterized by either urine output >0.5 ml/kg for 2-h or lactate decrease by >10%) in septic shock [6].

- 2. Early initiation of vasopressors can potentially increase cardiac output and improve tissue and organ perfusion by several mechanisms (Fig. 8.1).

  - Firstly, by its venoconstrictive effects norepinephrine can potentially recruit unstressed volume to stressed volume especially in patients with profound vasodilation, increase mean systemic filling pressure and increase venous return [7]. Same mechanism can explain possible synergistic effect of norepinephrine along with fluid bolus or infusion.
  - Secondly, norepinephrine can increase cardiac output by increasing cardiac contractility [8]. Two possible

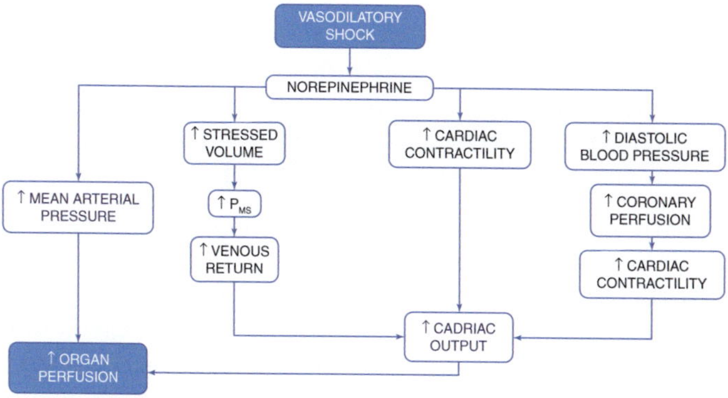


FIGURE 8.1 Possible mechanisms for improvement in organ perfusion by vasopressor infusion

explanations for this increase in cardiac contractility are beta-1 adrenergic stimulation of cardiomyocytes and increase in coronary perfusion pressure by an increase in diastolic blood pressure.

3. By increasing mean arterial pressure early norepinephrine administration recruit more microvessels, improve microcirculation and organ perfusion. This later mechanism is especially important for patients with profound hypotension.
   - In a prospective study of 28 patients with septic shock, an increase in MAP from 54 to 77 mmHg with norepinephrine infusion was shown to increase muscle tissue oxygen saturation ($StO_2$, an indirect reflection of microcirculation) significantly from 74% to 78%, along with a significant increase in cardiac index [9].
4. Cumulative fluid balance is a concerning point in acutely ill patients and higher balance is clearly shown to be associated with higher mortality [10]. Early norepinephrine infusion can potentially reduce total volume of resuscitation and cumulative fluid balance.
   - In multicentre REFRESH study, early administration of norepinephrine (after 1000 ml of resuscitation fluid) had shown to reduce both resuscitation volume and total infusion volume at both 6-h and 24-h after starting resuscitation, in patients with sepsis [11].
   - Early norepinephrine infusion has also been shown to reduce cumulative exposure to vasopressors potentially reducing their harmful effects [5, 11].
5. Early norepinephrine infusion can improve outcomes in sepsis including mortality [5], early resolution of shock, [6] reduction in incidence of pulmonary oedema or new-onset arrhythmias [6]. In a single-centre RCT, a strategy of norepinephrine infusion along with fluid infusion was shown to improve in-hospital mortality in septic shock (compared to a strategy of norepinephrine infusion only after 30 ml/kg fluid bolus) [12]. Despite these potential benefits, there are

still controversies regarding the generalizability of this strategy. There are also concerns about how to apply this strategy at the bedside [13]. Some simple rules may help in defining the timing of vasopressor (especially norepinephrine) in patients with septic shock.

1. Start norepinephrine infusion immediately in patients with low diastolic blood pressure (DBP <50 mmHg) or high diastolic shock index (heart rate / DBP >2.3) with or without evidence of hyperdynamic circulation (pulse pressure > 40 mmHg) [14].
2. Otherwise, start norepinephrine infusion after initial crystalloid boluses (say approximately 500–1000 ml) without waiting for 30 ml/kg bolus [11]. This recommendation is particularly relevant in patients with profound hypoxia.
3. In patients with low pulse pressure (<40 mmHg), it is however reasonable to give more emphasis on fluid infusion aiming to improve stroke volume.

## 8.3 Vasopressors: Classification

- Vasopressors can be classified based on their mechanisms of action and predominant receptors on which they act. A proposed classification system is depicted in Table 8.1. Predominant effect on a particular receptor may be dose-dependent.
- **Norepinephrine:**
  - By predominant alpha effect norepinephrine increase both venous and arterial tone, increases cardiac preload (by increasing venous return), arterial pressure and systemic vascular resistance.
  - By beta-mediated increase in cardiac contractility, it can increase cardiac output.
  - It produces baroreceptor-mediated reflex bradycardia (by increasing mean arterial pressure).

Table 8.1 Classification of commonly used vasopressors based on their effect on different receptors

| Drug | Dose | Alpha 1 | Beta 1 | Beta 2 | DOPA | V1 | V2 | AGT-R I/II |
|---|---|---|---|---|---|---|---|---|
| *Catecholamines* | | | | | | | | |
| Norepinephrine (mcg/kg/min) | 0.01–3 | ++++ | ++ | – | – | – | – | – |
| Epinephrine (mcg/kg/min) | 0.01–0.05 | + | +++ | ++ | – | – | – | – |
| | >0.05 | ++++ | ++ | ++ | – | – | – | – |
| Dopamine (mcg/kg/min) | 1–5 | – | + | – | ++++ | – | – | – |
| | 5–10 | + | ++ | – | +++ | – | – | – |
| | 10–20 | +++ | ++ | – | + | – | – | – |
| Phenylephrine (mcg/kg/min) | 0.4–9 | ++++ | – | – | – | – | – | – |
| *Vasopressin and analogues* | | | | | | | | |
| Vasopressin (unit/min) | 0.03–0.04 | – | – | – | – | ++++ | +++ | – |
| Terlipressin (mcg/kg/h) | 1.3 | – | – | – | – | V1a (V1b) | + | – |
| Selepressin (ng/kg/min) | 1.25–2.5 | – | – | – | – | V1a selective | – | – |
| *Angiotensin II receptor (AGT-R I/AGT-R II) agonists* | | | | | | | | |
| Angiotensin II (mcg/kg/min) | 5–2200 | – | – | – | – | – | – | ++++ |

- Potential adverse effects include cardiac arrhythmias, peripheral ischemia and inadvertent immunosuppression.

- **Epinephrine:**
  - In low doses, epinephrine increases cardiac contractility, increases heart rate and increases cardiac output, by its predominant effect on beta 1 receptor.
  - By beta 2 effect, it can also produce vasodilatation and some fall in MAP.
  - At higher doses, it increases venous and arterial tone by predominant alpha receptor effect.
  - It has significant effects on metabolism including stimulation of glycogenolysis and gluconeogenesis with resulting hyperglycaemia, aggravated further by increased insulin resistance (alpha effect). It can increase lipolysis and increase lactate production.
  - Potential adverse effects include tachycardias, tachyarrhythmias, metabolic adverse effects as discussed above, splanchnic and peripheral ischemia.

- **Dopamine:**
  - At low dose, acts predominantly on dopamine receptors, increases renal blood flow and produces an increase in urine output. However, this apparent "Renal Protective" effect of dopamine has not been substantiated in clinical studies.
  - It has predominantly beta 1 effects at moderate doses increasing cardiac contractility.
  - At higher doses, alpha effects predominate, producing vasoconstriction and rise in blood pressure.
  - Dopamine decreases serum concentrations of all anterior pituitary hormones including prolactin, thyrotrophic releasing hormone, growth hormone (GH, also disturbs normal pulsatile secretion of GH) and luteinizing hormone. It can also induce or aggravate sick euthyroid syndrome by suppressing secretion of thyroid-stimulating hormone and also by decreasing free T4 and T3 levels.

- Dopamine can also have immunosuppressive effects.
- Major adverse effects of dopamine include tachycardia, tachyarrhythmias, apart from its effects on the endocrine system and immunity (as described above).

- **Phenylephrine:**
  - Phenylephrine is not routinely used as a first-line vasopressor in acute care setting.
  - It is predominantly an alpha-adrenergic agonist with minimal beta activity and is a pure vasoconstrictor.
  - It increases systemic vascular resistance and mean arterial pressure, causes reflex bradycardia and reduces cardiac output by increasing afterload of left ventricle.
  - In 2011, amidst a nationwide shortage of norepinephrine in the USA, phenylephrine was the most commonly used alternative vasopressor for septic shock. An increase in septic shock mortality was noticed during the same period, raising a strong possibility of higher risk of death associated with the use of phenylephrine (compared to norepinephrine) in septic shock [15].

- **Vasopressin:**
  - Vasopressin is a hormone secreted from the supraoptic and paraventricular nuclei of hypothalamus and is stored in posterior pituitary. In a physiological state, it is released from posterior pituitary primarily in response to increased serum osmolality, but also during hypovolemia or in the presence of other stimuli, e.g. pain. In patients with sepsis, there is often a relative vasopressin deficiency.
  - Vasopressin acts on different receptors and produces a multitude of effects. By acting on V1a receptors, present in smooth muscle and myocardium, it causes vasoconstriction, increase in venous and arterial tone and also platelet aggregation. Stimulation of V1b receptors present in the central nervous system, increases secretion of corticotrophin-releasing hormone. V2 receptors (in collecting ducts and distal convoluted tubules of nephron)

stimulation is associated with water retention (discussed further in Chap. 2).
- Skin necrosis is common with extravasation of vasopressin and hence it should not be used through peripheral cannula.
- Other major adverse effects of vasopressin include digital, myocardial and mesenteric ischemia.

- **Terlipressin:**
  - Terlipressin is a relatively selective vasopressin analogue acting predominantly on V1a and V1b receptors producing vasoconstriction, increase in mean arterial pressure and increase in systemic vascular resistance.
  - In a multicentre RCT, terlipressin infusion failed to demonstrate any mortality benefit over norepinephrine infusion in septic shock. In the same study, terlipressin was associated with a significant increase in adverse effects [16].
  - Moreover, it may be difficult to titrate terlipressin infusion because of its prolonged half-life.
  - Terlipressin is not recommended for routine use as a vasopressor.

- **Selepressin:**
  - Selepressin is a selective V1a receptor agonist.
  - Initially, there was a lot of enthusiasm about this molecule, especially in septic shock, because of its potential role in reducing capillary leak, improving hemodynamic variables and reduction in mortality in animal models.
  - However, in a large multicentre SEPSIS-ACT study, it failed to demonstrate any outcome benefit compared to placebo, in patients with septic shock [17].
  - Selepressin is currently not recommended as a vasopressor.

- **Angiotensin II:**
  - AT-II is a non-adrenergic vasoconstrictor that can increase venous and arterial tone.

  - It can also increase ACTH, ADH and aldosterone levels.
  - Potential adverse effects of angiotensin II include tachycardia, peripheral ischemia and thromboembolic events.
  - ATHOS-3 study has convincingly demonstrated its benefit (compared to placebo) in increasing blood pressure in patients with vasodilatory shock who were not responding to conventional high-dose vasopressors [18].
  - However, till further data is available on patient-centric outcomes, use of angiotensin II should be limited to highly selective patients.

## 8.4 Which Vasopressor?

- Till date, no randomized trial has shown the mortality benefit of one vasopressor over another. Thus, the choice of vasopressor is currently based on their physiological role in different shock states, user experience, adverse event profile, convenience and cost.
- Pivotal clinical trials comparing different vasopressors are shown in Table 8.2.
- From the available evidence, the following recommendations can be made.
  - In patients with vasoplegic shock especially septic shock, norepinephrine should be the first-line vasopressor of choice [1].
  - In children, however, epinephrine may be considered as the first-line agent because of issues related to vascular access (as extravasation of norepinephrine from peripheral intravenous access can cause more tissue damage in children).
  - Vasopressin or epinephrine can be added as the second-line agent in non-responsive patients [1]. Vasopressin infusion should perhaps be started early (within 6–12 h of septic shock onset) and at a lower norepinephrine dose (<15 mcg/min) [21].

TABLE 8.2 Pivotal randomized trials comparing different vasopressors

| Trial | Patient | Intervention | Control | Primary outcome | Secondary outcome |
|---|---|---|---|---|---|
| CATS [19] | Multicentre RCT. Septic shock. N = 330 | Epinephrine titrated to maintain MAP >70 mmHg. | Norepinephrine titrated to maintain MAP >70 mmHg + Dobutamine (if needed). | No difference in 28-day mortality. | No between-group difference in efficacy and safety. |
| CAT [20] | Multicentre RCT. Patients requiring vasopressors. N = 208 | Epinephrine to achieve MAP ≥70 mmHg. | Norepinephrine to achieve MAP ≥70 mmHg. | No difference in median time to achieve MAP goal for >24 H without vasopressor. | No difference in 28-day or 90-day mortality. No difference in different subgroups of shock. *12.9% of patients in epinephrine group withdrew because of transient but significant metabolic side effects.* |

(continued)

Table 8.2 (continued)

| Trial | Patient | Intervention | Control | Primary outcome | Secondary outcome |
| --- | --- | --- | --- | --- | --- |
| VASST [21] | Multicentre RCT.<br>Septic shock on norepinephrine infusion.<br>N = 778 | Blinded infusion of low-dose vasopressin (0.01–0.03 U/min) in addition to open-label norepinephrine to achieve target MAP. | Blinded infusion of norepinephrine (5–15 mcg/min) in addition to open-label norepinephrine to achieve target MAP. | No difference in 28-day mortality. | No overall difference in serious adverse events.<br>*Lower 28-day mortality in vasopressin group, in pre-specified stratum of patients with less severe septic shock at baseline (norepinephrine infusion < 15 mcg/min)* |
| SOAP II [22] | Multicentre RCT.<br>Patients in shock requiring vasopressor.<br>N = 1679 | Dopamine infusion (up to 20 mcg/kg/min) to maintain BP. | Norepinephrine infusion (up to 0.19 mcg/kg/min) to maintain BP. | No difference in 28-day mortality. | *More arrhythmias in patients treated with dopamine.*<br>In subgroup of patients with cardiogenic shock, dopamine infusion was associated with increased 28-day mortality. |

| | | | | | |
|---|---|---|---|---|---|
| VANISH [23] | Multicentre RCT. Septic shock within 6-h of onset requiring vasopressor. N = 409 | Vasopressin infusion (titrated up to 0.06 U/min) PLUS either hydrocortisone or placebo. | Norepinephrine infusion PLUS either hydrocortisone or placebo. | No difference in kidney failure-free days at day-28. | No difference in 28-day mortality. Lower creatinine and higher urine output over first 7-days in vasopressin group. Lower RRT requirement in vasopressin group. No difference in serious adverse events. Mean dose norepinephrine and vasopressin on the day of serious adverse events were 0.55 mcg/kg/min and 0.06 U/min, respectively. |

*RCT* randomized control trial, *MAP* mean arterial pressure, *BP* blood pressure

- Dopamine should only be used in patients with bradycardia and hypotension [1].
- In patients with cardiogenic shock, norepinephrine should be the first-line vasopressor [22].
- In patients with hypovolemic and haemorrhagic shock, focus should be on correction of volume deficit and haemostatic resuscitation respectively PLUS correction of underlying defect (discussed in detail in Chaps. 12 and 13). Vasopressor infusion should be started only in life-threatening hypotension. Again, norepinephrine should possibly be the first-choice agent [22].

## 8.5 Blood Pressure Target

- Surviving Sepsis Campaign guidelines suggest an initial MAP target of 65–70 mmHg for patients with septic shock [1]. This recommendation is based on some small studies. One of these small studies showed, no differences in physiological variables including lactate, gastric mucosal $PaCO_2$ or hourly urine output when different MAP targets were set at 65 or 75 or 85 mmHg [24].
- However, many experts in the field argue that target MAP should be higher in some patients especially those with pre-existing chronic hypertension. Some others opine that, in elderly patients, MAP target should be lower, as they are at a higher risk of adverse consequences of vasopressors, including ischemic events or arrhythmias.
- Three well-designed randomized clinical trials have addressed the issue of high versus low MAP target and are summarized in Table 8.3.
- While choosing target blood pressure, balance must be made between maintaining perfusion by increasing upstream pressure for tissue perfusion (MAP) and adverse consequences of vasopressors including ischemia and arrhythmias. Following approach may be useful.
  - For most patients with vasodilatory shock initial blood pressure target may be MAP between 65 to 70 mmHg [1].

TABLE 8.3 Randomized clinical trials comparing higher versus lower mean arterial pressure (MAP) target

| | **SEPSISPAM study** [25] | **OVATION study** [26] | **65 study** [27] |
|---|---|---|---|
| Setting | Multicentre RCT. 29 French hospitals. | Multicentre pilot RCT. 11 academic centres from the USA and Canada. | Multicentre RCT. 65 ICUs from the United Kingdom. |
| Patients | Adult patients with septic shock. N = 776 | Adult patients with vasodilatory shock. N = 118 | 65 years or older patients with vasodilatory shock. N = 2600 |
| Intervention | Resuscitation targeting MAP 80–85 mmHg (high MAP Group) | Lower MAP target 60–65 mmHg. | MAP target 60–65 mmHg (permissive hypotension) |
| Control | Resuscitation targeting MAP 65–70 mmHg (low MAP Group) | Higher MAP target 75–80 mmHg. | Usual care. MAP target at the discretion of treating clinician. |
| Primary outcome | No difference in 28-day mortality. | Significant between-group separation in MAP. Mean difference of 9 mmHg. | No difference in unadjusted all-cause mortality at day-90. |

(continued)

TABLE 8.3 (continued)

| | **SEPSISPAM study** [25] | **OVATION study** [26] | **65 study** [27] |
|---|---|---|---|
| Secondary outcome | No difference in 90-day mortality or organ dysfunction. Higher incidence of new AF in high MAP Group. In patients with pre-existing chronic hypertension, high MAP Group had lower doubling of creatinine and lower need for RRT. | No difference in ICU, in-hospital or 28-day mortality. No difference in cardiac arrhythmias. No difference in renal SOFA score changes. No outcome differences in subgroup of patients with chronic hypertension. In patients 75 years or older, low MAP target was associated with lower in-hospital mortality. | Permissive hypotension group received significant lower duration of vasopressor and lower dose of norepinephrine equivalent. After adjusting for pre-specified baseline variables, there was a small but significant difference in 90-day mortality favouring permissive hypotension group. No difference in serious adverse events. |

However, in patients 65 years or older a lower target MAP of 60 to 65 mmHg is safe and perhaps beneficial [27].

– Patients whose tissue perfusion is not maintained with this initial target MAP PLUS adequate fluid resuscitation, MAP may be increased to 85 to 90 mmHg for a short duration by increasing vasopressor dose ("**Vasopressor Challenge**") [28]. If the tissue perfusion is improved with this new MAP target, patients should continue with the new target. If the perfusion does not improve, vasopressor infusion should be reduced to achieve the lower target set earlier. The later strategy

was used in ANDROMEDA-SHOCK study but was limited to patients with pre-existing chronic hypertension [29].
 – In patients with haemorrhagic shock, initial blood pressure target should be much lower before achieving haemostasis to avoid an increase in bleeding unless there is an associated head injury (discussed further in Chap. 12).

## 8.6 Case Scenario (Continued)

- Mr. VG is in septic shock with very low DBP and has already received 1-Litre of intravenous fluid. He is also significantly hypoxemic.
- Starting norepinephrine infusion at this stage will not only help in restoring his MAP early but also will improve the coronary perfusion pressure by restoring DBP. This will potentially limit the cumulative resuscitation volume and avoid worsening of hypoxemia.
- Initial MAP target should be 60 to 70 mmHg.
- Further fluid boluses should be planned cautiously keeping in mind aggravation of hypoxemia and only if he remains hypoperfused with evidence of fluid responsiveness (discussed in Chap. 9).
- If the hypoperfusion persists despite reaching the initial MAP target and after adequate fluid resuscitation "vasopressor challenge" may be considered to look for individualized MAP target.

**Take-Home Messages**

- In life-threatening hypotension vasopressor infusion must be started immediately—before or along with fluid resuscitation. Even otherwise, starting vasopressor early has several advantages.
- Norepinephrine is the vasopressor of choice in most clinical situations.

- In vasoplegic shock, vasopressin should be added early as the second agent if the norepinephrine infusion rate is escalating rapidly.
- Initial MAP target for vasopressor infusion should be between 60 and 65 mmHg. But the target must be individualized keeping in mind the ultimate goal of organ perfusion.

## References


1. Evans L, Rhodes A, Alhazzani W, Antonelli M, Coopersmith CM, French C, et al. Surviving sepsis campaign: international guidelines for management of sepsis and septic shock 2021. Intensive Care Med. 2021;2:1–67.
2. Scheeren TWL, Bakker J, De Backer D, Annane D, Asfar P, Boerma EC, et al. Current use of vasopressors in septic shock. Ann Intensive Care. 2019;9:20.
3. Brunauer A, Koköfer A, Bataar O, Gradwohl-Matis I, Dankl D, Dünser MW. The arterial blood pressure associated with terminal cardiovascular collapse in critically ill patients: a retrospective cohort study. Crit Care. 2014;18:719.
4. Karpati PC, Rossignol M, Pirot M, Cholley B, Vicaut E, Henry P, et al. High incidence of myocardial ischemia during postpartum hemorrhage. Anesthesiology. 2004;100:30–6.
5. Bai X, Yu W, Ji W, Lin Z, Tan S, Duan K, et al. Early versus delayed administration of norepinephrine in patients with septic shock. Crit Care. 2014;18:532.
6. Permpikul C, Tongyoo S, Viarasilpa T, Trainarongsakul T, Chakorn T, Udompanturak S. Early use of norepinephrine in septic shock resuscitation (CENSER). A randomized trial. Am J Respir Crit Care Med. 2019;199:1097–105.
7. Persichini R, Silva S, Teboul JL, Jozwiak M, Chemla D, Richard C, Monnet X. Effects of norepinephrine on mean systemic pressure and venous return in human septic shock. Crit Care Med. 2012;40:3146–53.
8. Hamzaoui O, Jozwiak M, Geffriaud T, Sztrymf B, Prat D, Jacobs F, et al. Norepinephrine exerts an inotropic effect during the early phase of human septic shock. Br J Anaesth. 2018;120:517–24.

9. Georger JF, Hamzaoui O, Chaari A, Maizel J, Richard C, Teboul JL. Restoring arterial pressure with norepinephrine improves muscle tissue oxygenation assessed by near-infrared spectroscopy in severely hypotensive septic patients. Intensive Care Med. 2010;36:1882–9.
10. Boyd JH, Forbes J, Nakada TA, Walley KR, Russell JA. Fluid resuscitation in septic shock: a positive fluid balance and elevated central venous pressure are associated with increased mortality. Crit Care Med. 2011;39:259–65.
11. Macdonald SPJ, Keijzers G, Taylor DM, Kinnear F, Arendts G, Fatovich DM, et al. Restricted fluid resuscitation in suspected sepsis associated hypotension (REFRESH): a pilot randomised controlled trial. Intensive Care Med. 2018;44:2070–8.
12. Elbouhy MA, Soliman M, Gaber A, Taema KM, Abdel-Aziz A. Early use of norepinephrine improves survival in septic shock: earlier than early. Arch Med Res. 2019;50:325–32.
13. Waechter J, Kumar A, Lapinsky SE, Marshall J, Dodek P, Arabi Y, et al. Interaction between fluids and vasoactive agents on mortality in septic shock: a multicenter, observational study. Crit Care Med. 2014;42:2158–68.
14. Ospina-Tascón GA, Teboul JL, Hernandez G, Alvarez I, Sánchez-Ortiz AI, Calderón-Tapia LE, et al. Diastolic shock index and clinical outcomes in patients with septic shock. Ann Intensive Care. 2020;10:41.
15. Vail E, Gershengorn HB, Hua M, Walkey AJ, Rubenfeld G, Wunsch H. Association between US norepinephrine shortage and mortality among patients with septic shock. JAMA. 2017;317:1433–42.
16. Liu ZM, Chen J, Kou Q, Lin Q, Huang X, Tang Z, et al. Terlipressin versus norepinephrine as infusion in patients with septic shock: a multicentre, randomised, double-blinded trial. Intensive Care Med. 2018;44:1816–25.
17. Laterre PF, Berry SM, Blemings A, Carlsen JE, François B, Graves T, et al. Effect of selepressin vs placebo on ventilator- and vasopressor-free days in patients with septic shock: the SEPSIS-ACT randomized clinical trial. JAMA. 2019;322:1476–85.
18. Khanna A, English SW, Wang XS, Ham K, Tumlin J, Szerlip H, et al. Angiotensin II for the treatment of vasodilatory shock. N Engl J Med. 2017;377:419–30.
19. Annane D, Vignon P, Renault A, Bollaert PE, Charpentier C, Martin C, et al. Norepinephrine plus dobutamine versus epinephrine alone for management of septic shock: a randomised trial. Lancet. 2007;370:676–84.

20. Myburgh JA, Higgins A, Jovanovska A, Lipman J, Ramakrishnan N, Santamaria J, CAT Study Investigators. A comparison of epinephrine and norepinephrine in critically ill patients. Intensive Care Med. 2008;34:2226–34.
21. Russell JA, Walley KR, Singer J, Gordon AC, Hébert PC, Cooper DJ, et al. Vasopressin versus norepinephrine infusion in patients with septic shock. N Engl J Med. 2008;358:877–87.
22. De Backer D, Biston P, Devriendt J, Madl C, Chochrad D, Aldecoa C, et al. Comparison of dopamine and norepinephrine in the treatment of shock. N Engl J Med. 2010;362:779–89.
23. Gordon AC, Mason AJ, Thirunavukkarasu N, Perkins GD, Cecconi M, Cepkova M, et al. Effect of early vasopressin vs norepinephrine on kidney failure in patients with septic shock: the VANISH randomized clinical trial. JAMA. 2016;316:509–18.
24. LeDoux D, Astiz ME, Carpati CM, Rackow EC. Effects of perfusion pressure on tissue perfusion in septic shock. Crit Care Med. 2000;28:2729–32.
25. Asfar P, Meziani F, Hamel JF, Grelon F, Megarbane B, Anguel N, et al. High versus low blood-pressure target in patients with septic shock. N Engl J Med. 2014;370:1583–93.
26. Lamontagne F, Meade MO, Hébert PC, Asfar P, Lauzier F, Seely AJE, et al. Higher versus lower blood pressure targets for vasopressor therapy in shock: a multicentre pilot randomized controlled trial. Intensive Care Med. 2016;42:542–50.
27. Lamontagne F, Richards-Belle A, Thomas K, Harrison DA, Sadique MZ, Grieve RD, et al. Effect of reduced exposure to vasopressors on 90-day mortality in older critically ill patients with vasodilatory hypotension: a randomized clinical trial. JAMA. 2020;323:938–49.
28. Coimbra KTF, de Freitas FGR, Bafi AT, Pinheiro TT, Nunes NF, Nathaly F, et al. Effect of increasing blood pressure with noradrenaline on the microcirculation of patients with septic shock and previous arterial hypertension. Crit Care Med. 2019;47:1033–40.
29. Hernández G, Ospina-Tascón GA, Damiani LP, Estenssoro E, Dubin A, Hurtado J, et al. Effect of a resuscitation strategy targeting peripheral perfusion status vs serum lactate levels on 28-day mortality among patients with septic shock: the ANDROMEDA-SHOCK randomized clinical trial. JAMA. 2019;321:654–64.

# Part III
# Useful Concepts to Understand

# Chapter 9
# Concept of Fluid Responsiveness. Fluid Challenge

## 9.1 Case Vignette

Mr. DG, a 74-year-old male with history of long-standing diabetes mellitus, hypertension and nephropathy is admitted with fever and cough for last 3 days. On examination, he is confused with heart rate 112/min regular, non-invasive blood pressure 84/46 mmHg, respiratory rate 30/min and $SpO_2$ of 96% on 4 litres of $O_2$. Clinical examination is consistent with left-sided pneumonia and evidence of circulatory shock. Blood gas shows: pH 7.36, $PaO_2$ 64 mmHg (on 4 litres $O_2$), $PaCO_2$ 32.8 mmHg, $HCO_3^-$ 19.2 mmol/L. Serum lactate is 4.6 mmol/L. He has already received 1500 ml of Ringer's Lactate in the Emergency Department.

### *9.1.1 What should be the Most Rational Strategy for Fluid Administration after Initial Bolus?*

Deciding the need for volume expansion is one of the biggest therapeutic dilemmas faced by an acute care physician. This may not be a big issue in the very early stage of resuscitation with obvious hypovolemia. However, once the patient has already received significant volume of fluid during the process of resuscitation, further fluid therapy has the potential to



S. Ghosh, *Handbook of Intravenous Fluids*,
https://doi.org/10.1007/978-981-19-0500-1_9

produce volume overload with associated morbidity and mortality. On the other hand, not giving fluid to a patient who may benefit from it can compromise tissue perfusion further. In this situation, clinicians have two options to resolve this issue:

- Perform some clinical manoeuvres or observe certain clinical parameters to predict effect of further fluid on cardiac output, also known as "**Fluid Responsiveness**".
- Actually, administer a measured volume of fluid rapidly under close monitoring and look for its effect on cardiac output or its surrogate, also known as "**Fluid Challenge**".

In this chapter, we shall discuss different tests to predict fluid responsiveness, appropriate use of these tests in clinical scenarios and their limitations. We shall also discuss the right technique for performing a fluid challenge.

## 9.2 Fluid Responsiveness

- Some hemodynamic parameters detected during clinical monitoring or manipulated in certain ways have shown to predict response of fluid infusion on cardiac output. These fluid responsiveness parameters can be classified into— "**Static**" and "**Dynamic**" parameters.
  - **Static Indices:** These are the stand-alone measurements of cardiac preload or surrogate parameters. Examples include central venous pressure (CVP), pulmonary artery occlusion pressure (PAOP), left ventricular end-diastolic volume (LVEDV, measured by echocardiography), global end-diastolic volume (GEDV, measured by thermodilution technique), etc. There is now a large body of literature available, confirming the futility of these static parameters in predicting response to fluid infusion with reasonable accuracy. Hence, their use should be abandoned for this purpose.
  - **Dynamic Indices:** These are the manoeuvres that test the current position of the patient in his or her cardiac

function curve, by taking advantage of respiratory variations in preload parameters or by changes in preload condition utilizing the patient's own preload reserve. Dynamic indices are considered to be more accurate measures for predicting fluid responsiveness.

## 9.3 Respirophasic Variations in Pulse Pressure

- Phasic variations of stroke volume (cardiac output), systolic pressure and pulse pressure during positive pressure ventilation are described in Chap. 3 and can be utilized for predicting fluid responsiveness in an appropriate clinical context.
- **Pulse Pressure Variation:** The physiological principle behind pulse pressure variation is shown in Fig. 9.1, with lower panel showing changes in airway pressure during controlled positive pressure breathing in volume control mode and upper panel showing arterial pressure tracing. Baseline pulse pressure can be measured by applying an end-expiratory pause.

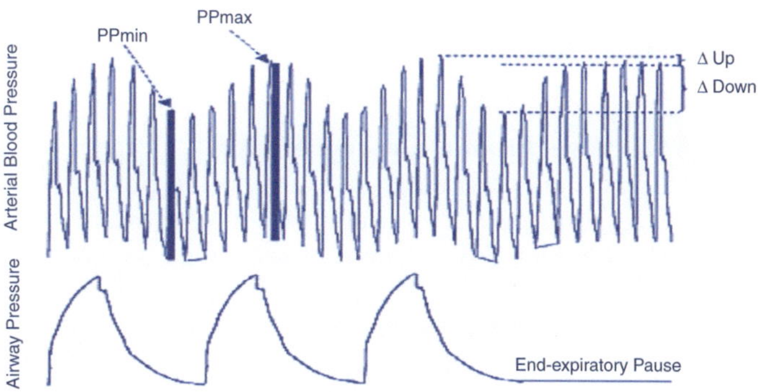


FIGURE 9.1 Simultaneous recording of airway pressure and arterial pressure tracings during positive pressure ventilation

- As can be seen, pulse pressure is maximum at the peak of inspiratory pressure rise (PPmax) and lowest during expiration (PPmin).
  - Maximum pulse pressure observed during positive pressure inspiration is because of simultaneous rise of left ventricular pre-load (parallel ventricular interdependence and squeeze effect on pulmonary veins) and decrease in LV afterload.
  - Decrease in LV preload (because of series ventricular interdependence) and increased LV afterload during expiration, result in low pulse pressure.
- The difference between PPmax and PPmin is known as pulse pressure variation which clearly has two different components (**ΔUp**, difference between PPmax and baseline PP) and (**ΔDown**, difference between PP and PPmin).
  - **ΔUp** component is more prominent in patients with LV dysfunction.
  - Whereas in patients with absolute or relatively depleted intravascular volume, **ΔDown** component becomes exaggerated.
  - Exaggerated pulse pressure variation in intravascular volume-depleted patients (predominantly because of **ΔDown** effect) can be utilized for predicting fluid responsiveness (see Box 9.1).

**Box 9.1 PPV—Proof of Concept Study** [1]

- Michard and colleagues investigated the predictive ability of respiratory variation of pulse pressure on response to volume challenge in 40 mechanically ventilated patients with septic shock.
- They calculated pulse pressure variation as the difference between PPmax and PPmin in one respiratory cycle divided by the mean of these two.

$$\mathrm{PPV} = \left(\mathrm{PP}_{\mathrm{max}} - \mathrm{PP}_{\mathrm{min}}\right) \times 100 / \mathrm{Mean\ of\ PP}_{\mathrm{max}}\ \mathrm{and\ PP}_{\mathrm{min}})$$

- The study concluded that in appropriately selected mechanically ventilated patients with circulatory shock, pulse pressure variation can differentiate between fluid responders and non-responders.
- With a cut-off value of 13%, it has a sensitivity of 94% and specificity of 96% in predicting fluid responsiveness.

- However, Pulse Pressure Variation (PPV) has several limitations and it is valid only in mechanically ventilated patients. Some of the important limitations of PPV are enumerated in Table 9.1.

TABLE 9.1 Limitations of PPV and other tests of fluid responsiveness based on principles of heart–lung interaction

| Condition | Limitation | Mechanism |
|---|---|---|
| Spontaneous breathing effort | False-positive | By exaggerating pleural and intrathoracic pressure changes. |
| Cardiac arrhythmias | False-positive | Because of variation in duration of diastole with higher stroke volume post longer diastole and vice versa. |
| Low VT, <8 ml/kg predicted body wt. | False-negative | Reduction in amplitude of change in pleural pressure. |
| Severe ARDS with low lung compliance | False-negative | By reducing transmission of intra-alveolar pressure to intravascular and intra-cardiac compartments. |
| Open chest | False-negative | Inability to contain changes in pleural and intrathoracic pressure. |
| Increased intra-abdominal pressure | False-positive | Exaggerated respiratory variation in intrathoracic pressure changes. PPV may still be useful with higher threshold value. |

(continued)

Table 9.1 (continued)

| Condition | Limitation | Mechanism |
|---|---|---|
| Very high respiratory rate (HR/RR <3.6) | False-negative | Effect of decreased RV stroke volume during positive pressure inspiration only transmits to the left side after 3–4 heartbeats, producing decreased LV preload during expiration.<br>With high RR, the next respiratory cycle starts early without manifesting decreased LV preload effect. |
| Right heart failure | False-positive | Increase afterload of right ventricle limiting RV stroke volume further in RV failure overall exaggerating ΔDown component. |

## 9.4 Systolic Pressure Variation (SPV) and Stroke Volume Variation (SVV)

- Both these tests use the same principle as PPV, with similar limitations as described in Table 9.1.

## 9.5 Respiratory Variations of Vena Caval Diameter

- Intrathoracic pressure changes during positive pressure breath may induce some changes in the diameter of venae cavae in close proximity to the heart. This effect is exaggerated in the presence of relative or absolute hypovolemia.
- **Inferior Vena Cava (IVC) Distensibility:** IVC can be visualized in the sub-xiphoid view using transthoracic echocardiography and its diameter can be measured in M-mode just upstream of the origin of hepatic vein.

- IVC diameter increases with an increase in intrathoracic pressure during positive pressure inspiration.
- IVC distensibility index (dIVC) is the reflection of this increase in diameter during positive pressure inspiration and can be calculated as (See Box 9.2):

$$\frac{\text{Maximum diameter on inspiration} - \text{Minimum diameter on expiration}}{\text{Minimum diameter on expiration}}$$

- IVC Distensibility shares same limitations as PPV and is not valid in spontaneously breathing patients.

**Box 9.2 IVC Distensibility—Proof of Concept Study** [2]

- Validity of dIVC was tested in 23 mechanically ventilated septic shock patients without any spontaneous breathing effort.
- The study found dIVC as an accurate predictor of fluid responsiveness.
- With a cut-off value of 18%, it had a sensitivity of 90% and a specificity of 90% in predicting fluid responsiveness.

- **Superior Vena Cava (SVC) Collapsibility:** Superior Vena Cava (SVC) can be visualized by trans-oesophageal echocardiography.
  - Being an intrathoracic structure, SVC collapses during positive pressure inspiration and it bounces back during expiration.
  - SVC Collapsibility, i.e. the percentage of decrease in SVC diameter during inspiration can be calculated as (see Box 9.3):

$$\frac{\text{Maximum diameter on expiration} - \text{Minimum diameter on inspiration}}{\text{Maximum diameter on expiration}}$$

**Box 9.3 SVC Collapsibility—Proof of Concept Study** [3]
- In appropriately selected patients in circulatory shock, superior vena cava collapsibility was found to discriminate between patients who will respond to fluid bolus ("Fluid responders") and who will not ("Fluid Non-responders") with reasonable accuracy.
- SVC collapsibility cut-off value of 36% had a sensitivity of 90% and a specificity of 100% for predicting fluid responsiveness.

- The accuracy of SVC collapsibility index is found to be marginally superior to IVC distensibility index in predicting fluid responsiveness, but the test itself is limited by the need for trans-oesophageal echocardiography [4]. This test also has same limitations as PPV or IVC distensibility.

## 9.6 End-Expiratory Occlusion Test

- Positive pressure insufflation during mechanical ventilation impedes the venous return and in turn decreases cardiac pre-load and cardiac output. Interrupting mechanical insufflation at the end of expiration for a few seconds can interrupt this cycle and increase the cardiac pre-load transiently.
  - For a measurable increase in cardiac output, this end-expiratory occlusion (EEO) must be for at least 15 s, as this is the minimal time required for the right-sided pre-load change to transmit to the left-side through pulmonary circulation.
  - Increase in cardiac output following 15 s EEO is more prominent in hypovolemic patients. Hence, this manoeuvre can be utilized to differentiate between fluid responders and non-responders in a mechanically ventilated patients in circulatory shock [5, see Box 9.4].

- Some key points regarding EEO are given below.
  - EEO has the advantage of being a simple manoeuvre.
  - Its ability to predict fluid responsiveness remains valid even in patients of ARDS (with low compliance) on low tidal volume ventilation and in the presence of arrhythmias.
  - Real-time cardiac output measurement during the procedure is preferred while performing the test. However, in the absence of CO monitoring increase in pulse pressure during end-expiratory pause can be taken as a useful surrogate. An increase in End-tidal Carbon Di-oxide ($ETCO_2$) with 15-second end-expiratory occlusion can also be considered as a surrogate of cardiac output monitoring during this manoeuvre.
  - Increase in aortic velocity time integral (VTI) in transthoracic echocardiography can also be used in place of real-time cardiac output monitoring during EEO. However, limitations of echocardiography (including its operator dependence and difficulties in measuring VTI in emergency situations) must be kept in mind while recommending this as a surrogate of cardiac output during EEO.
  - The test is obviously limited by its inability to be useful in non-intubated patients.
  - Its value is also limited in patients who are breathing very rapidly and who cannot tolerate 15-s end-expiratory hold.

**Box 9.4 EEO—Proof of Concept Study** [5]
- In 34 mechanically ventilated, who were planned to receive fluid bolus, Monnet and colleagues performed 15-s end-expiratory occlusion test before actually loading them with fluid.
- Fluid responsiveness could be predicted by demonstrating an increase in pulse pressure by >5% during the end-expiratory occlusion with sensitivity and a specificity of 87% and 100%, respectively.

## 9.7 Passive Leg Raising

- Passive leg raising (PLR) acts on the principle of "**Auto-Fluid Challenge**" by mobilizing approximately 300 ml of blood from lower half of the body to the central circulation and by monitoring its effect on cardiac output or its surrogate.
- Advantages of this test are its documented validity even in spontaneously breathing patients and in patients with arrhythmias or ARDS. But to get an accurate result, following rules must be followed while performing the test [6].

1. Any activity that can evoke sympathetic response like touching the patient, coughing or manually raising the end of the bed must be avoided. Respiratory secretion must be cleared carefully using gentle suctioning prior to performing the test. Lower end of the bed must be elevated using an automated system.
2. Since PLR-induced changes in cardiac output are short-lasting (<1 min), cardiac output must be monitored with a real-time monitoring.
    - Aortic blood flow monitoring by oesophageal Doppler or $ETCO_2$ monitoring can be used as surrogate of cardiac output during passive leg raise [6, 7].
    - Utility of changes in pulse pressure as a surrogate of cardiac output monitoring during passive leg raising is limited because the manoeuvre itself can modulate the amplification of pulse waves [8]. However, in resource-limited settings change in pulse pressure following passive leg raising can still be utilized to predict fluid responsiveness. With a threshold of increase in pulse pressure by 10%, it has a pooled sensitivity of 62% and specificity of 83% in predicting fluid responsiveness [9].
3. Raising legs from supine position can only recruit blood volume from lower limbs. However, making the trunk horizontal from a semi-recumbent position (as shown in

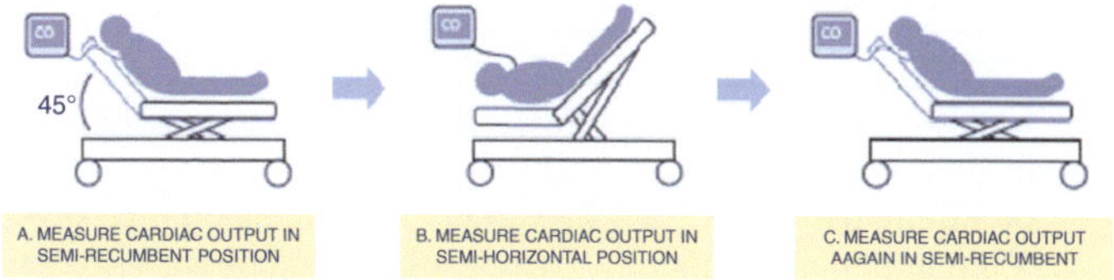


FIGURE 9.2 Passive leg raising test

Fig. 9.2) can additionally recruit volume from splanchnic circulation.

- Hence, initially, patients should be positioned 45-degree semi-recumbent for obtaining baseline measurement (Fig. 9.2A).
- Next, the bed should be adjusted to make the trunk parallel to the floor (with lower limbs at 45 degrees now) and cardiac output measurement is repeated in less than 1-min time (Fig. 9.2B).
- Cardiac output should be measured again after moving the patient back to semi-recumbent position to see whether the same returns back to baseline (Fig. 9.2C). Later measurement is performed to ensure that the change in cardiac output during PLR manoeuvre is actually because of auto-fluid challenge, not simply because of the spontaneous changes inherent to the underlying disease process.

4. 10% increase in cardiac output (by real-time cardiac output monitor) [7, 10, see Box 9.5] or its surrogate like aortic blood flow (by oesophageal Doppler) or a 5% increase in $ETCO_2$ [8] predicts fluid responsiveness.

   - More recently some researchers have suggested a decrease in capillary refill time by 27% following passive leg raising as a predictor of fluid responsiveness [11]. However, it may be practically too difficult to measure such a tiny change in capillary refill time.

5. PLR has its own limitations. Advantages and limitations of PLR manoeuvre in predicting fluid responsiveness are summarized in Table 9.2.

Table 9.2 Passive leg raising: advantages and disadvantages

| Advantages | Limitations |
|---|---|
| 1. Can be performed in spontaneously breathing patients.<br>2. Valid in patients with arrhythmias.<br>3. Usefulness remains even in patients on low tidal volume ventilation and patients with low lung compliance. | 1. Needs real-time cardiac output monitoring.<br>2. Validity in patients on high-dose vasopressors and/or with severe hypovolemia is doubtful.<br>3. Not valid in patients with high intra-abdominal pressure.<br>4. Technical difficulties in patients with unstable spinal injury or fractured pelvis.<br>5. Contra-indicated in raised intracranial pressure. |

**Box 9.5 PLR—Proof of concept study** [10]

- Monnet and colleagues studied the accuracy of PLR manoeuvre in predicting fluid responsiveness in 71 mechanically ventilated patients with preserved spontaneous breathing with or without arrhythmias.
- They could demonstrate that PLR induced increase in aortic blood flow (a surrogate of cardiac output) by ≥10% predicts fluid responsiveness with a sensitivity of 97% and specificity of 94%.
- PLR induced increase in pulse pressure by ≥12% also found to predict fluid responsiveness but with a significantly lower sensitivity of 60% and a reasonable specificity of 85%.

## 9.8 Fluid Challenge

- In certain clinical circumstances, it may be difficult to utilize tests for fluid responsiveness, either because of limitations of the test itself or because of non-availability of appropriate resources. Validated fluid challenge test may be useful in deciding further fluid therapy in these situations.

- Fluid challenge can be defined as a technique to test preload responsiveness of circulatory system by rapid administration of defined volume of fluid to stretch the right side of the heart, looking for significant increase in stroke volume post-fluid challenge. A negative or positive fluid challenge lets the clinician take a decision regarding further administration of fluid.
- The fluid challenge technique we discuss in this chapter was described originally by Weil and Henning in 1979 [12]. More recently this concept was by Vincent and Weil in 2006 [13].

  – It starts with identifying clinical triggers from history, physical examination and routine laboratory values suggesting possible benefits of improving cardiac output in a particular patient. By themselves, these triggers do not have sufficient sensitivity or specificity to predict response to fluid infusion. Trigger for fluid challenge may be mottled skin, prolonged capillary refill time, tachycardia, low blood pressure, low urine output, raised serum lactate, etc.
  – With the recognition of appropriate trigger, a provocative test is initiated by rapidly infusing a defined volume of fluid looking for any increase in cardiac output, while constantly monitoring its effect on ventricular filling pressure.
  – This fluid challenge technique has four components and is described below. A useful pneumonic suggested by original authors to remember these four components is **T-R-O-L** [12, 13].

- **Type of fluid**: Both crystalloid and colloid can be utilized for fluid challenge. However, in most clinical situations some isotonic balanced crystalloid is preferred. Important points to remember are:

  – Hypotonic fluid should not be used.
  – Colloids do not have any specific advantage in most clinical situations and are costlier.

- Synthetic colloids especially hydroxyethyl starch have harmful consequences on kidneys, coagulation and reticuloendothelial system and can potentially increase mortality.
- Albumin is safe and may be considered in patients with hypoalbuminemia.
- Balanced crystalloids have some advantages over 0.9% Saline in most clinical situations except in patients with raised intracranial pressure.

- **Rate of fluid**: The volume and rate of infusion should be sufficient to stretch the system and increase mean systemic pressure.
  - A pharmacodynamic study of fluid challenge by Aya and colleagues suggested a volume of at least 4 ml/kg body weight given over 5 min as the minimal volume required to increase the mean systemic pressure [14].
  - Usual recommended rate is 500 ml crystalloid or 250 ml of colloid over 15 min.

- **Objective:** The objective of fluid challenge is to see an increase in cardiac output by at least 15% after the challenge (defined as "Fluid Responders").
  - Monitors must have the ability to identify small changes in cardiac output in real time. Thermodilution cardiac output measurements (intermittent or semi-continuous) may not be fast enough to guide fluid challenge.
  - When real-time cardiac output monitor is not available, other surrogate measures can be used. Example: aortic flow velocity from oesophageal Doppler or aortic root velocity time integral (VTI) from apical 4-chamber echocardiographic view.
  - In resource-limited setting, changes in arterial pressures can be utilized as a surrogate of cardiac output. An increase in pulse pressure or PP by 17% correlates best with an increase in cardiac output by >15% with a sensitivity of 65% and specificity of 85% [15]. Considering changes in Mean arterial pressure and diastolic blood

pressure as surrogate of cardiac output may result in large number of false-negative fluid challenges [15].
   - An ongoing clinical trial is testing feasibility of a fluid challenge induced decrease in CRT in predicting the need for further fluid (AUSTRALIS, Clinical trial registration no NCT04693923).
   - Changes in urine output or lactate cannot be taken as an objective for fluid challenge because of their slow change.

- **Limit:** The inherent limitation of fluid challenge is an increase in filling pressure leading to undesirable systemic or pulmonary oedema. This can be avoided by continuously monitoring filling pressure and putting some safety limits on it as suggested by Weil and Henning in their original paper.

   - Central venous pressure should be measured continuously during fluid challenge. At 10 min if the CVP remains below <2 mmHg, the infusion should be continued. If the CVP increased by 2 to 5 mmHg, the infusion should be interrupted temporarily and to be re-started only if it reduces after 10 min of wait. If the change in CVP is by >5 mmHg at any time the infusion must be stopped ("2 to 5" rule).
   - Similar stoppage rule is applicable for pulmonary artery occlusion pressure and is called the "3 to 7" rule.
   - Other safety limits could be by actually looking for pulmonary oedema (but only after it has already developed) and stopping the fluid infusion with its earliest evidence. Development of pulmonary oedema can be monitored clinically or by lung ultrasound (appearance of B-lines in anterior chest) or by measurement of extravascular lung water or by chest X-ray.

- Table 9.3 describes two examples of Fluid challenge technique as described above.
- **Limitations of Fluid Challenge:** The technique described above is logistically limited by relatively poor sensitivity of

TABLE 9.3 Example of a typical fluid challenge with two possible results

| **Mr. DG. Pneumonia. Septic shock. PP 38 mmHg. CVP 8 mmHg.** | **Example 1** | | | **Example 2** | | |
|---|---|---|---|---|---|---|
| **Plan: Fluid Challenge** | **Baseline** | **+10 min** | **+ 20 min** | **Baseline** | **+10 min** | **+20 min** |
| Type of fluid? Ringer's lactate | | | | | | |
| Rate of fluid? 500 ml over 15 min. | | | | | | |
| Objective? PP >45 mmHg | PP 38 | PP 42 | PP 48 | PP 38 | PP 40 | PP 43 |
| Safety limit? CVP 11 mmHg | CVP 8 | CVP 9 | CVP 10 | CVP 8 | CVP 10 | CVP 12 |
| | | Continue | Stop | | Continue | Stop |
| | Successful fluid challenge | | | Unsuccessful fluid challenge | | |

*PP* pulse pressure, *CVP* central venous pressure

non-invasive measures to be used as a surrogate of cardiac output monitoring.

- Another bigger limitation is that in addition to being a test, fluid challenge is a treatment on its own.
- Unsuccessful fluid challenge (possible in 50% of situation) has the potential to produce haemodilution, an increase in filling pressure and volume overload [16]. In hemodynamically unstable patients requiring 4- or 5-times fluid challenge in a day, this volume overload may be quite substantial!!
- Following measures may help in avoiding this volume overload:

1. Do not repeat the fluid challenge if the initial challenge is negative. Use some other ways to look for response to fluids or start (escalate) vasopressor [17].
2. Challenge the patient with smaller fluid volume more rapidly ("Mini-Fluid Challenge" described in the next section) [18].

## 9.9 Mini-Fluid Challenge

- There are some suggestions for performing fluid challenges with small volume of fluid up to 50–100 ml to avoid excess fluid overload (see Box 9.6).
- But as expected, the change in preload and cardiac output produced by this "mini"-fluid challenge is minimal and often short-lasting. Thus, concept of mini-fluid challenge requires very accurate real-time cardiac output monitoring.
- Unfortunately, the technique itself still lacks wide acceptance in acute care community.

**Box 9.6 Mini-fluid challenge—proof of concept study** [18]

- Muller and colleagues, studied the ability of "mini-fluid challenge" in predicting fluid responsiveness in 39 critically ill patients. 100 ml hydroxyethyl starch was infused over 1 min and change in subaortic velocity time index (VTI) was measured using trans-thoracic echocardiography.
- Change in VTI by >10% following 100 ml mini-fluid challenge predicted fluid responsiveness with a sensitivity and specificity of 95% and 78%, respectively and an area under the receiver operating characteristic curve of 0.92.

## 9.10 Case Scenario (Continued)

- In the given case scenario, with Mr. DG having already received 1.5 litres of fluid and being hypoxic, fluid responsiveness should be checked before administering further fluid infusion.
- Since he is not intubated, PLR induced change in cardiac output should be the most appropriate test for checking fluid responsiveness status.
- However, if real-time cardiac output monitoring is not available or in a busy emergency department scenario, a carefully performed fluid challenge test (as described above) could also be appropriate.

**Take-Home Messages**

- Fluids are drugs with definite risk of overdose (fluid overload). Need for fluid administration must be established with reasonable accuracy before its administration.
- Predictors of fluid responsiveness are useful in limiting fluid overload.

- All tests for fluid responsiveness have significant limitations. Appropriateness of a particular test should be based on the condition of patient and the availability of a particular test. A scheme for choosing appropriate tests for fluid responsiveness is given in Fig. 9.3. Sometimes a combination of tests may be useful.
- In a significant number of acutely ill patients, none of the tests for fluid responsiveness may be applicable. A carefully performed fluid challenge test may be useful in such cases.
- Fluid challenge should not be repeated if the initial test is negative or equivocal.

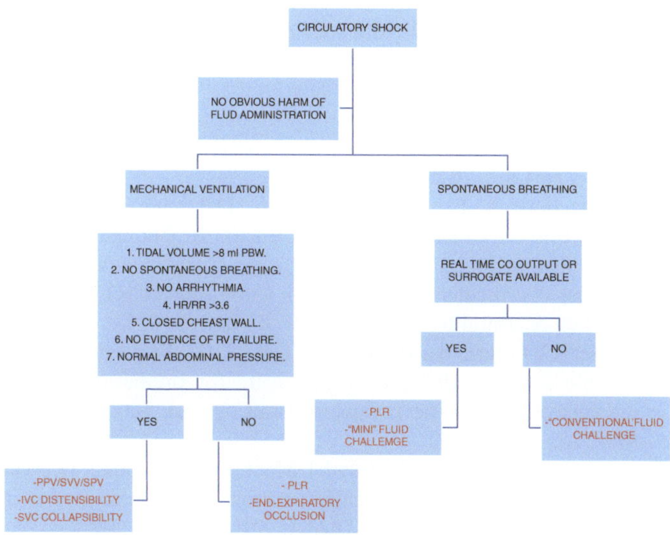


FIGURE 9.3 A Decision tree to apply tests for fluid responsiveness

## References

1. Michard F, Boussat S, Chemla D, Anguel N, Mercat A, Lecarpentier Y, et al. Relation between respiratory changes in arterial pulse pressure and fluid responsiveness in septic patients with acute circulatory failure. Am J Respir Crit Care Med. 2000;162:134–8.
2. Barbier C, Loubières Y, Schmit C, Hayon J, Ricôme JL, Jardin F, Vieillard-Baron A. Respiratory changes in inferior vena cava diameter are helpful in predicting fluid responsiveness in ventilated septic patients. Intensive Care Med. 2004;30:1740–6.
3. Vieillard-Baron A, Chergui K, Rabiller A, Peyrouset O, Page B, Beauchet A, Jardin F. Superior vena caval collapsibility as a gauge of volume status in ventilated septic patients. Intensive Care Med. 2004;30:1734–9.
4. Charbonneau H, Riu B, Faron M, Mari A, Kurrek MM, Ruiz J, et al. Predicting preload responsiveness using simultaneous recordings of inferior and superior vena cavae diameters. Crit Care. 2014;18:473.
5. Monnet X, Osman D, Ridel C, Lamia B, Richard C, Teboul JL. Predicting volume responsiveness by using the end-expiratory occlusion in mechanically ventilated intensive care unit patients. Crit Care Med. 2009;37:951–6.
6. Monnet X, Teboul JL. Passive leg raising: five rules, not a drop of fluid! Crit Care. 2015;19:18.
7. Lafanechère A, Pène F, Goulenok C, Delahaye A, Mallet V, Choukroun G, Chiche JD, Mira JP, Cariou A. Changes in aortic blood flow induced by passive leg raising predict fluid responsiveness in critically ill patients. Crit Care. 2006;10:R132.
8. Monnet X, Bataille A, Magalhaes E, Barrois J, Le Corre M, Gosset C, Guerin L, Richard C, Teboul JL. End-tidal carbon dioxide is better than arterial pressure for predicting volume responsiveness by the passive leg raising test. Intensive Care Med. 2013;39:93–100.
9. Bentzer P, Griesdale DE, Boyd J, MacLean K, Sirounis D, Ayas NT. Will this hemodynamically unstable patient respond to a bolus of intravenous fluids? JAMA. 2016;316:1298–309.
10. Monnet X, Rienzo M, Osman D, Anguel N, Richard C, Pinsky MR, Teboul JL. Passive leg raising predicts fluid responsiveness in the critically ill. Crit Care Med. 2006;34:1402–7.
11. Jacquet-Lagrèze M, Bouhamri N, Portran P, Schweizer R, Baudin F, Lilot M, Fornier W, Fellahi JL. Capillary refill time varia-

tion induced by passive leg raising predicts capillary refill time response to volume expansion. Crit Care. 2019;23:281.
12. Weil MH, Henning RJ. New concepts in the diagnosis and fluid treatment of circulatory shock. Thirteenth annual Becton, Dickinson and Company Oscar Schwidetsky memorial lecture. Anesth Analg. 1979;58:124–32.
13. Vincent JL, Weil MH. Fluid challenge revisited. Crit Care Med. 2006;34:1333–7.
14. Aya HD, Ster IC, Fletcher N, Grounds RM, Rhodes A, Cecconi M. Pharmacodynamic analysis of a fluid challenge. Crit Care Med. 2016;44:880–91.
15. Monnet X, Letierce A, Hamzaoui O, Chemla D, Anguel N, Osman D, Richard C, Teboul JL. Arterial pressure allows monitoring the changes in cardiac output induced by volume expansion but not by norepinephrine. Crit Care Med. 2011;39:1394–9.
16. Michard F, Teboul JL. Predicting fluid responsiveness in ICU patients: a critical analysis of the evidence. Chest. 2002;121:2000–8.
17. Cecconi M, Hofer C, Teboul JL, Pettila V, Wilkman E, Molnar Z, et al. Fluid challenges in intensive care: the FENICE study: a global inception cohort study. Intensive Care Med. 2015;41:1529–37.
18. Muller L, Toumi M, Bousquet PJ, Riu-Poulenc B, Louart G, Candela D, et al. AzuRéa group. An increase in aortic blood flow after an infusion of 100 ml colloid over 1 minute can predict fluid responsiveness: the mini-fluid challenge study. Anesthesiology. 2011;115:541–7.

# Chapter 10
# Four Phases of Fluid Resuscitation

## 10.1 Case Scenario

Mrs. AG, a 50-year-old woman presented to the ED with a stab injury to her abdomen. On examination, she was sweating profusely with cold extremities, heart rate 124/min and blood pressure 76/46 mmHg. FAST examination revealed free fluid in right superior quadrant with evidence of liver laceration. After 1000 ml of warm Ringer's lactate, she was taken up for laparotomy. Massive transfusion protocol was initiated. In the operation theatre, she received 6 units of packed RBCs, 6 units of fresh frozen plasma and 6 units of platelets plus additional 1500 ml of RL. Following peritoneal toilet, packing of liver and colostomy, she was shifted to ICU. On examination in the ICU, she is now under the effect of general anaesthesia, mild hypothermic, body temperature 96°F, heart rate 108/min, blood pressure 110/68 mmHg on low-dose norepinephrine infusion.

### *10.1.1 Does the Fluid Strategy vary in Different Stages of Resuscitation?*

Pathophysiology of circulatory shock is a dynamic process, with changes observed at both macro- and microcirculatory



S. Ghosh, *Handbook of Intravenous Fluids*,
https://doi.org/10.1007/978-981-19-0500-1_10

levels and in the metabolic milieu. These dynamic changes result both from the treatment provided and from human being's robust compensatory response to injury including inflammatory response as well as endocrine changes. Response to fluid therapy, both beneficial and potentially harmful, depends on which phase of circulatory shock the patient is in. In this chapter, we shall discuss different phases of circulatory shock and the potential role of fluid in each phase. However, these phases described in this chapter are only conceptual and not mutually exclusive. Patients can move from one phase to another in each direction and may skip a phase completely.

## 10.2 Four-Hit Model of Circulatory Shock

- Way back in 1942, Cuthbertson described two phases of metabolic response to injury [1].
- He described an initial phase called "**Ebb Phase**" characterized by arterial underfilling and dysfunction of microcirculation resulting from true hypovolemia (from disease process itself) or relative hypovolemia due to vasodilatation, capillary leak (and interstitial oedema) resulting from the release of inflammatory cytokines.
  - Ebb phase results in hypoperfusion and impaired tissue oxygenation.
  - This phase is characterized by hypothermia, low oxygen consumption, lactic acidosis, increased production and release of stress hormones, decreased release of insulin, increased gluconeogenesis, hyperglycaemia, increased consumption of substrates, immune activation and increased hepatic acute phase response.
- Cuthbertson also described a second phase, called "**Flow Phase**" that developed within 48–72 h, if the patient survives the initial insult.
  - Flow phase is an anabolic phase that results from restoration of flow to the organs and is characterized by features exactly the reverse of ebb phase.

- More recently, Malbrain and colleagues described a Three-Hit model of circulatory and metabolic derangement following an acute insult, based on a retrospective analysis of data from their ICU [2, 3]. The model is illustrated in Fig. 10.1 (adapted from Reference [3]).

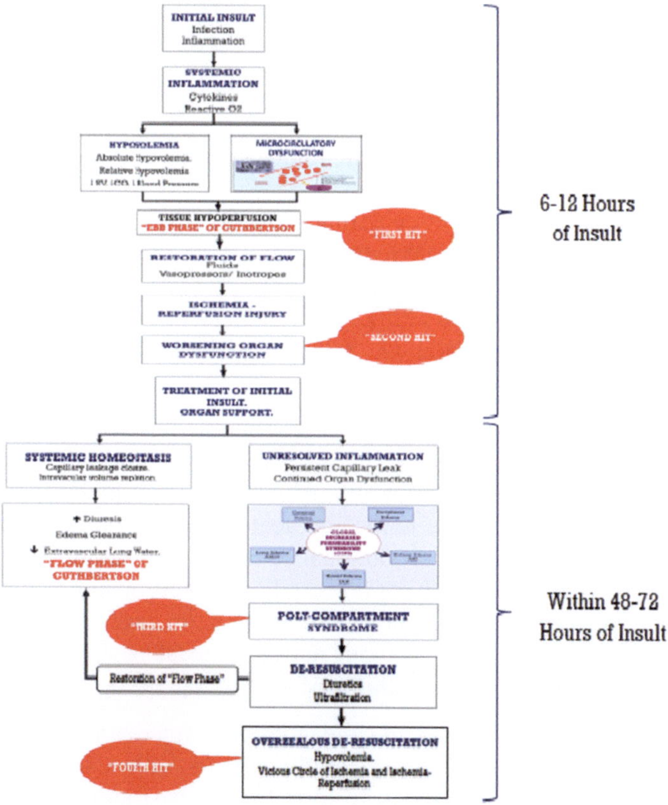


FIGURE 10.1 Four-Hit model of circulatory shock. *CO* cardiac output, *GIPS* global increased permeability syndrome, *ARDS* acute respiratory distress syndrome, *IAH* intra-abdominal hypertension, *AKI* acute kidney injury

- Hypovolemia, either true or relative (due to vasodilatation and capillary leak), from initial insult results in tissue injury because of hypoperfusion, much the same way as described in the ebb phase of Cuthbertson ("**First Hit**").
  - At this stage, an aggressive fluid resuscitation can restore the flow at a cost of reperfusion-related injury to the tissue and organs ("**Second Hit**"). First and second hit usually occurs within 6–12 h of insult.
- Over the next 3 days, capillary leak is repaired, macrocirculation as well as microcirculatory parameters show improvement, and systemic homeostasis is restored (flow phase of Cuthbertson).
- But in some patients, inflammatory processes remain unresolved with persistent leaky capillaries resulting in interstitial oedema, aggravated further by intravascular volume expansion ("**Third Hit**"). Malbrain and colleagues termed this later condition as "**Global Increased Permeability Syndrome**" (GIPS).
  - GIPS results in poly-compartment syndrome—lung oedema or acute respiratory distress syndrome, brain oedema, raised intra-abdominal pressure, compartment syndrome of the limbs and acute kidney injury due to renal oedema or abdominal compartment syndrome.
  - GIPS can be either prevented or treated by more conservative fluid management in the later stages of resuscitation with or without active removal of fluid (also known as de-resuscitation).
- Years ago, Murphy and colleagues performed a retrospective cohort study of 212 adult patients with acute lung injury and septic shock to look for the best approach to managing fluid in these patients [4]. Logical conclusion of the study (that fits into the Three-Hit model just described) was that a fluid management strategy targeting both adequate initial fluid resuscitation (AIFR) and conservative late fluid management (CLFM) can achieve maximum survival advantage (Fig. 10.2) [4].

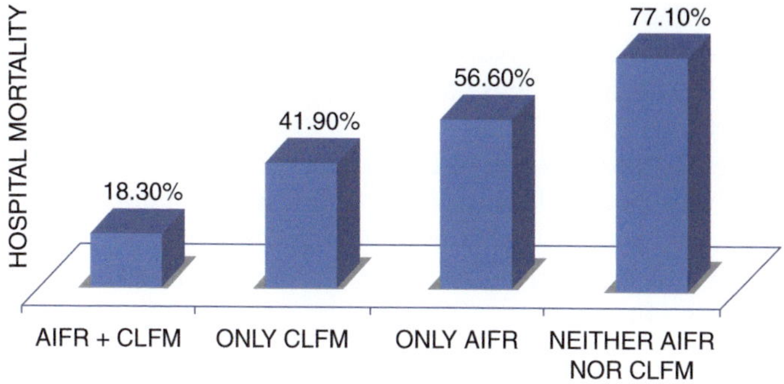


FIGURE 10.2 Aggressive early resuscitation and late conservative strategy achieves best mortality outcome. *AIFR* aggressive initial fluid resuscitation, *CLFM* conservative late fluid management

- Murphy and colleagues arbitrarily defined AIFR as fluid bolus of at least 20 ml/kg bolus before initiating vasopressors with a CVP goal >8 mmHg within 6 h of septic shock onset (just for understanding the concept not to take this definition letter and spirit!) and CLFM as even to negative fluid balance for at least 2 consecutive days in the first 7 days after sepsis onset.

- Malbrain and colleagues went on to add a "**Fourth Hit**" concept to their model [5]. This fourth hit can result from an overzealous prescription of de-resuscitation measures that can lead to hypovolemia and repetition of the whole cycle.

## 10.3 4-Phases of Fluid Resuscitation

- Based on the discussion above, we can now decipher four distinct (but dynamic) phases of fluid resuscitation: Resuscitation (or Rescue) Phase, Optimization Phase, Stabilization Phase and Evacuation Phase (acronym R-O-S-E, famous "**ROSE**" concept) [5].

- Other authors named these phases somewhat differently as: Salvage Phase, Optimization Phase, Stabilization Phase and De-escalation Phase (acronym S-O-S-D) [6, 7].

- **Resuscitation Phase:** In this phase, also known as rescue or salvage phase, fluid is given as boluses to rapidly correct hypovolemia with a goal to achieve minimal cardiac output and blood pressure to sustain life (taking care of the "First Hit").
  - In this phase, patients are monitored clinically with peripheral perfusion markers, blood pressure, heart rate, level of sensorium, lactate, etc.
  - At the end of this phase (no definite way to define but possibly after initial fluid boluses or maybe within 3–6 h of the onset of shock) the patient is in positive fluid balance.
- **Optimization Phase:** In this phase, patients are at compensatory shock, either following initial resuscitation or due to patients' own homeostatic response and are no longer at imminent life-threatening state.
  - The goal of fluid therapy at this stage is to optimize cardiac output further without worsening re-perfusion injury (taking care of "Second Hit").
  - This is achieved by giving small fluid boluses, provided the patient is still fluid responsive or by monitored fluid challenge, at the same time avoiding any harm resulting from fluid therapy.
  - This phase requires more sophisticated monitoring including tests for fluid responsiveness, cardiac output monitoring in selected patients and careful monitoring for extravascular fluid accumulation by lung ultrasound or extravascular lung water.
  - Decision to infuse fluid at this phase also should consider the appropriate clinical context like ongoing volume loss due to diarrhoea or harm of continuing fluid in a patient with pneumonia and severe hypoxemia.

- **Stabilization Phase:** In this phase, patient is not in circulatory shock or impending shock, requiring only maintenance fluid to cater to the obligatory requirement of the body or replacement fluid to correct ongoing volume loss.
  - Goal is to keep the patient euvolemic. Any positive fluid balance will contribute to worsening of the organ function (taking care not to initiate "Third Hit").
  - One should not forget fluid infused through medication or as flush solutions (termed as "Fluid Creep" by some researchers [8]) while calculating maintenance fluid need.
  - If everything goes well, patient shows signs of recovery over the next 2–3 days.
- **Evacuation Phase:** From the discussion earlier, we now know that some patients continue to show evidence of capillary leak even during stabilization phase and develop global increased permeability syndrome.
  - GIPS is further aggravated by positive fluid balance in stabilization phase. A strategy of "**late goal-directed fluid removal**" may be beneficial in such patients [3, 9, 10]. The term "**De-resuscitation**" is coined to describe this process of fluid removal and is widely used today in the field of intravenous fluid therapy [10, 11].
  - In the next section, we shall be discussing the science behind and the art of de-resuscitation process.

## 10.4 De-resuscitation

- De-resuscitation can be defined as a strategy of forceful fluid removal in addition to conservative fluid management strategy in the late stage of resuscitation, in patients who are hemodynamically stable, aiming to prevent (and treat) end-organ damage resulting from fluid overload.
- Malbrain and colleagues have defined "**Fluid Overload**" as cumulative fluid balance exceeding 10% of patients baseline body weight (Cumulative fluid balance in litre/Patient's baseline body weight × 100) [11].

  - When it is not measured routinely, baseline body weight can be substituted by ideal body weight.

- There are a number of publications on the efficacy of de-resuscitation measures and these are summarized in Table 10.1. However, there are significant limitations of all these published studies:

  - Heterogeneity of the study designs
  - Small number of patients enrolled
  - Heterogeneity of patient population studied
  - Different inclusion criteria used
  - Different end-point used

- Despite these limitations, all of them have shown consistent benefits associated with de-resuscitation measures, confirming the data from observational studies [10]. More importantly, de-resuscitation measures were found to be safe with no increase in systemic adverse events, when performed in a controlled manner.
- **De-resuscitation in practice:** Questions that need to be answered during de-resuscitation process are: When to initiate? How to initiate? What to monitor? When to stop?
- **When to initiate?** De-resuscitation should be initiated if there is evidence of fluid overload as defined earlier with or without obvious tissue oedema, e.g. pedal oedema, ascites, raised intra-abdominal pressure, several B-lines in multiple lung zones or increased extravascular lung water, etc. But before that patient must be hemodynamically stable, not requiring additional fluid boluses or replacement fluids and no or minimal dose of vasopressors.
- **How to initiate?** Fluid removal can be done either by judicious use of diuretics or by ultrafiltration using continuous renal replacement therapy (CRRT) or by slow low-efficiency haemodialysis (SLED) when CRRT is not available.

  - One approach, as suggested by Berthelsen and colleagues, is to start with a 40 mg IV bolus of furosemide followed by infusion titrated to a maximum dose of 40 mg/h [15]. Alternatively, one may use torsemide.

Table 10.1 Summary of studies looking for the efficacy and safety of De-resuscitation Measures

| First author | Patient | Intervention | Control | Outcome |
|---|---|---|---|---|
| Martin GS et al. [12] Randomized control trial. 2 university hospitals from France. | ARDS. On MV. Total protein ≤5 gm/dl. N = 37 | Forced fluid removal with 25 gm albumin q 8-h PLUS furosemide infusion for 5 days. | No forced fluid removal. Dual placebo. | - 5.3 kg higher weight loss in intervention group compared to control.<br>- Improvement in PaO2/FIO2 ratio in intervention group.<br>- Favourable trend towards in ICU measures in intervention group. |
| Martin GS et al. [13] Randomized control trial. 2 university hospitals from France. | ARDS. On MV. Total protein ≤6 gm/dl. No hemodynamic instability or severe renal/hepatic failure. N = 40 | Forced fluid removal with furosemide infusion PLUS albumin. | Forced fluid removal with furosemide infusion PLUS placebo. | - Greater improvement in PaO2/FIO2 ratio in intervention group at 24 h and at Day 3.<br>- Higher net fluid loss in intervention group on Day 3.<br>- More hypotensive episodes and lower shock-free days in control group. |

(continued)

Table 10.1 (continued)

| First author | Patient | Intervention | Control | Outcome |
|---|---|---|---|---|
| Cordemans et al. [9] Retrospective matched, case-control study. Single centre from Belgium. | ARDS. On MV. Negative fluid balance deemed necessary in view of low PaO2/FIO2 ratio, high EVLWI and raised IAP.<br>N = 114 | Forced fluid removal with PAL approach:<br>**P**EEP matching IAP.<br>Small volume Hyperoncotic **a**lbumin<br>Fluid remova**l**—Diuresis or ultrafiltration. | None. | - Lower cumulative fluid balance and EVLWI at 7 days in PAL group.<br>- PAL group had higher PaO2/FIO2 ratio at 7 days.<br>- Higher 28-day survival in PAL group.<br>- No worsening cardiovascular or renal SOFA score at 7-days in PAL group. |
| Ganter CC et al. [14] Single-centre, single-arm feasibility study. | Sepsis or other inflammatory condition. On MV. AKI. With no substantial negative fluid balance following standard approach.<br>N = 10 | Protocolized fluid management strategy with CRRT for 3 days.<br>Close hemodynamic monitoring. | | - Higher fluid removal rate during study period compared to 3 days before.<br>- Overall there was no significant instability during study period with some adjustment in fluid removal rate. |

| | | | | |
|---|---|---|---|---|
| Berthelsen RE et al. [15]<br>Multicentre RCT.<br>Pilot study looking for feasibility of a larger study. | ICU patients with AKI and fluid accumulation of more than 10% IBW.<br>N = 23 | Protocolised forced fluid removal with furosemide infusion and/or CRRT aiming at net negative fluid balance >1 mL/kg ideal body weight/hour until cumulative fluid balance calculated from ICU admission reached <1000 ml. | Standard care.<br>CRRT discouraged unless absolutely indicated. | - Trial stopped prematurely after 20 months because of slow recruitment rate.<br>- Significantly higher negative fluid balance at Day 5 in intervention group.<br>- No increase in harm associated with forced fluid removal. |

(continued)

Table 10.1 (continued)

| First author | Patient | Intervention | Control | Outcome |
|---|---|---|---|---|
| Wang L et al. [16] Quasi-experimental, before and after study. Single Chinese centre. | Adult patients. Post-elective or emergency surgery. Shock requiring >1000 ml fluid infusion. >2000 ml cumulative fluid balance post-surgery. N = 85 | Fluid removal once the patient did not require any fluid bolus and large dose norepinephrine (<0.3 mcg/kg/min).<br>PLUS<br>Any two of the following four:<br>(i) IVC diameter ≥ 2 cm.<br>(ii) IVC diameter increased by ≥0.5 cm.<br>(iii) Significant changes in IVC diameter during respiration.<br>(iv) B-line positive region ≥1.<br>Fluid removal guided similarly by USG guidance with reversal of above parameters. | Fluid removal as per clinical experience. | - Forced fluid removal was started earlier, completed quicker and ended earlier in intervention group.<br>- Significantly higher daily negative fluid balance and urine output in intervention group.<br>- Shorter time of lung B-lines to reduction to zero was shorter in intervention group.<br>- Trend towards reduction in ICU-LOS in intervention group. |

*ARDS* acute respiratory distress syndrome, *MV* mechanical ventilation, *AKI* acute kidney injury, *EVLWI* extravascular lung water index (a measure of lung fluid accumulation), *CRRT* continuous renal replacement therapy, *USG* ultrasonography, *SOFA* sequential organ failure assessment

- CRRT or SLED should be considered in cases of inadequate response to diuretic or in anuric patients or in patients requiring renal replacement therapy for some other reason or in patients who developed serious adverse effects to furosemide or torsemide (e.g. thrombocytopenia, agranulocytosis, pancreatitis, life-threatening arrhythmias related to electrolyte disturbances, Steven Johnsons syndrome, toxic epidermal necrolysis, etc).
- Addition of hyperoncotic albumin boluses (or as infusion) produces significant increase in the rate of fluid removal [13]. One suggested approach is to infuse 100 ml boluses of 20 or 25% Albumin every 8-h (as 60-min intravenous infusion). Alternatively, 20 or 25% albumin may be administered as a continuous infusion at 20 ml/h.

• **What to monitor?** Patient should be monitored closely for any evidence of hypovolemia or hypoperfusion and adequacy of fluid removal. Goal should be to achieve a net negative fluid balance of at least 1 mL/kg IBW/h [15].

  - Patients should also be monitored for serious adverse effects of diuretics and electrolyte abnormalities e.g. hypokalaemia, dysnatremia, hypomagnesemia or hypophosphatemia.

• **When to stop?** De-resuscitation should be stopped or at least temporarily suspended if the patient fulfils any of the following criteria.

  - Circulatory instability as reflected by fall in blood pressure or need for up titrating vasopressor infusion, evidence of skin hypoperfusion e.g. mottling beyond the edge of kneecap or prolonged capillary refill time and unexplained elevation of lactate (especially if the value is >4 mmol/L). In that case, fluid removal must be suspended and fluid may be re-administered judiciously. Fluid removal may be re-initiated in a lower rate, once hypovolemia or hypoperfusion is mitigated.
  - Goal of slightly negative or zero fluid balance is achieved.

## 10.5 Case Scenario (Continued)

- Mrs. AG seems to be in the optimization phase with compensated shock following major haemorrhage.
- Post adequate control of haemorrhage, it is now time to look for evidence of fluid responsiveness and whether there is any potential harm associated with further fluid boluses.
  - She is at a high risk of developing intra-abdominal hypertension (and possible abdominal compartment syndrome) requiring careful monitoring of intra-abdominal pressure, in addition to monitoring for perfusion and fluid responsiveness.
  - She is also at a high risk of secondary ARDS, requiring careful monitoring of extravascular lung water and appearance of multiple B-lines in lung ultrasound.
- After the optimization phase, it will be important to maintain strict euvolemia in the stabilization phase.
- She may require active de-resuscitation, if negative balance is not achieved spontaneously between day 3 and day 7.

**Take-Home Messages**

- These are summarized in Fig. 10.3.

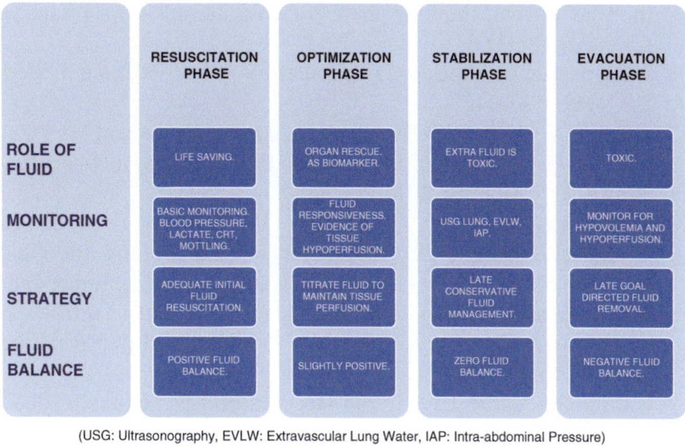


FIGURE 10.3 Stages of fluid resuscitation. *USG* ultrasonography, *EVLW* extravascular lung water, *IAP* intra-abdominal pressure

# References


1. Cuthbertson DP. Post-shock metabolic response. Lancet. 1942;1:433–7.
2. Malbrain MLNG, Regenmortel NV. Fluid overload is not only of cosmetic concern. ICU Management. 2012;1:30–3.
3. Cordemans C, De Laet I, Van Regenmortel N, Schoonheydt K, Dits H, Huber W, Malbrain MLNG. Fluid management in critically ill patients: the role of extravascular lung water, abdominal hypertension, capillary leak, and fluid balance. Ann Intensive Care. 2012;2(Supplement 1):S1.
4. Murphy CV, Schramm GE, Doherty JA, Reichley RM, Gajic O, Afessa B, Micek ST, Kollef MH. The importance of fluid management in acute lung injury secondary to septic shock. Chest. 2009;136:102–9.
5. Malbrain MLNG, Van Regenmortel N, Saugel B, De Tavernier B, Van Gaal PJ, Joannes-Boyau O, et al. Principles of fluid management and stewardship in septic shock: it is time to consider

the four D's and the four phases of fluid therapy. Ann Intensive Care. 2018;8(1):66.
6. Vincent JL, De Backer D. Circulatory shock. N Engl J Med. 2013;369:1726–34.
7. Hoste EA, Maitland K, Brudney CS, Mehta R, Vincent JL, Yates D, et al. Four phases of intravenous fluid therapy: a conceptual model. Br J Anaesth. 2014;113:740–7.
8. Van Regenmortel N, Verbrugghe W, Roelant E, Van den Wyngaert T, Jorens PG. Maintenance fluid therapy and fluid creep impose more significant fluid, sodium, and chloride burdens than resuscitation fluids in critically ill patients: a retrospective study in a tertiary mixed ICU population. Intensive Care Med. 2018;44:409–17.
9. Cordemans C, De Laet I, Van Regenmortel N, Schoonheydt K, Dits H, Martin G, Huber W, Malbrain ML. Aiming for a negative fluid balance in patients with acute lung injury and increased intra-abdominal pressure: a pilot study looking at the effects of PAL-treatment. Ann Intensive Care. 2012;2(Suppl 1):S15.
10. Silversides JA, Fitzgerald E, Manickavasagam US, Lapinsky SE, Nisenbaum R, Hemmings N, et al. Deresuscitation of patients with iatrogenic fluid overload is associated with reduced mortality in critical illness. Crit Care Med. 2018;46:1600–7.
11. Malbrain ML, Marik PE, Witters I, Cordemans C, Kirkpatrick AW, Roberts DJ, Van Regenmortel N. Fluid overload, deresuscitation, and outcomes in critically ill or injured patients: a systematic review with suggestions for clinical practice. Anaesthesiol Intensive Ther. 2014;46:361–80.
12. Martin GS, Mangialardi RJ, Wheeler AP, Dupont WD, Morris JA, Bernard GR. Albumin and furosemide therapy in hypoproteinemic patients with acute lung injury. Crit Care Med. 2002;30:2175–82.
13. Martin GS, Moss M, Wheeler AP, Mealer M, Morris JA, Bernard GR. A randomized, controlled trial of furosemide with or without albumin in hypoproteinemic patients with acute lung injury. Crit Care Med. 2005;33:1681–7.
14. Ganter CC, Hochuli R, Bossard M, Etter R, Takala J, Uehlinger DE, Jakob SM. Forced fluid removal in critically ill patients with acute kidney injury. Acta Anaesthesiol Scand. 2012;56:1183–90.

15. Berthelsen RE, Perner A, Jensen AK, Rasmussen BS, Jensen JU, Wiis J, Behzadi MT, Bestle MH. Forced fluid removal in intensive care patients with acute kidney injury: the randomised FFAKI feasibility trial. Acta Anaesthesiol Scand. 2018;62:936–44.
16. Wang L, Qiu C, Guan X, Chen M, Chen J, Si X, Du Z, Liu Y, Ouyang B. Fluid removal with ultrasound guided protocol improves the efficacy and safety of dehydration in post-resuscitated critically ill patients: a quasi-experimental, before and after study. Shock. 2018;50:401–7.

# Part IV
# Fluid Management in Specific Situations

# Chapter 11
# Fluid Resuscitation in Septic Shock

## 11.1 Case Vignette

Mr. AA, a 74-year-old gentleman with past history of Diabetes Mellitus and nephropathy presented to the ED with 3-days history of fever, cough and progressive breathlessness. On examination, he is confused with regular heart rate of 112/min, blood pressure 82/42 mmHg, respiratory rate 30/min and $SpO_2$ of 96% on 4 litres of $O_2$ by nasal prong. His hands are cool to touch with grossly delayed capillary refill time. Lung auscultation revealed bronchial breathing in left infrascapular and left axillary region suggestive of consolidation. Arterial blood gas showed pH 7.36, $PO_2$ 64 mmHg (on 4 litres $O_2$), $PaCO_2$ 32.8 mmHg, $HCO_3^-$ 19.2 mmol/L and lactate 4.6 mmol/L. ED physician is aware of the latest surviving sepsis guideline recommending rapid intravenous crystalloid bolus for initial resuscitation of Mr. AA.



S. Ghosh, *Handbook of Intravenous Fluids*,
https://doi.org/10.1007/978-981-19-0500-1_11

### *11.1.1 How Best to Resuscitate a Patient with Septic Shock?*

Circulatory shock is a life-threatening condition characterized by inadequate delivery of substrates to the tissues. The shock state is produced by individual defects at the level of macro- or micro-circulation or because of the loss of coherence between macro- and micro-circulation. Many decades ago, Weil and Shubin described four broad categories of shock, based on defects in macro-circulation—**Hypovolemic**, **Cardiogenic**, **Obstructive** and **Distributive** [1]. Septic shock, a type of distributive shock, is one of the leading causes of mortality and morbidity worldwide [2]. Recent consensus guideline defines sepsis as life-threatening organ dysfunction resulting from dysregulated host response to infection and septic shock as a subset of sepsis characterized by profound circulatory, cellular and metabolic abnormalities with a high risk of mortality [3].

In this chapter, we shall briefly discuss how effectively septic shock can be recognized at the bedside and how to apply diagnostic tools to understand the underlying source of infection. We shall also discuss in greater detail the principles of septic shock resuscitation.

## 11.2 Pathophysiology of Septic Shock

- Conventionally, pathophysiology of shock is explained by the mismatch between delivery of oxygen to the tissues and its extraction. Despite the lack of sound experimental evidence behind it, this traditional view still remains popular amongst acute care physicians, because of its simplicity and practicality.
- **Global delivery of oxygen (DO2)** is conceptualized as the total amount of oxygen delivered to the whole body in a minute and is determined by the **Cardiac Output** (CO, a product of stroke volume and heart rate per minute) and **Oxygen Content of the Arterial Blood** ($C_aO_2$).

- $DO_2 = CO \times C_aO_2$
- $C_aO_2 = (Hb \times S_aO_2 \times 1.34) + (P_aO_2 \times 0.003)$ (Where, Hb = Haemoglobin in gm/dl, $SaO_2$ = Oxygen saturation of haemoglobin, $PaO_2$ = Partial pressure of oxygen in arterial blood in mmHg.)
- Dissolved $O_2$ being negligible the equation can be simplified further. $DO_2 = CO \times (Hb \times S_aO_2 \times 1.34)$

- **Global consumption of oxygen (VO2)** is defined as the total amount of oxygen extracted by the body in a minute for aerobic metabolism. Mathematically global oxygen consumption is the product of cardiac output and the difference between arterial oxygen content ($CaO_2$) and the **Mixed Venous Oxygen Content** ($C_vO_2$, venous oxygen content in the pulmonary venous blood).
  - $VO_2 = CO \times (C_aO_2 - C_vO_2)$
  - $CvO_2 = (Hb \times S_vO_2 \times 1.34) + (P_vO_2 \times 0.003)$ (Where, $S_vO_2$ = Mixed venous oxygen saturation or saturation of pulmonary arterial blood, $P_vO_2$ = Partial pressure of oxygen in pulmonary arterial blood)
  - Once again, dissolved $O_2$ being negligible the equation can be modified further. $VO_2 = CO \times Hb\ X\ (S_aO_2 - S_vO_2) \times 1.34$
  - Under normal resting conditions with preserved cardiac output, adequate haemoglobin and adequate oxygen saturation of haemoglobin, $DO_2$ is more than adequate to meet $VO_2$.

- **Oxygen extraction ratio (O2ER)** is the ratio of oxygen consumption ($VO_2$) to oxygen delivery ($DO_2$) and can be calculated from the formula given below.
  - $O_2ER = VO_2/DO_2 = CO \times Hb \times (S_aO_2 - S_vO_2) \times 1.34/CO \times (Hb \times S_aO_2 \times 1.34$
    - $= (S_aO_2 - S_vO_2)/S_aO_2$
  - Interestingly $O_2ER$ of different tissues are not the same and varies from less than 15% in kidneys to more than 60% in heart.
  - In normal resting state, global $O_2ER$ is approximately 25%. During exercise, it can increase to as high as 75%.

- Till a certain value of $DO_2$ (called **Critical DO2**), utilization of oxygen in the tissues (or $VO_2$) remains independent of oxygen delivery.
  - This is possible, because of the adaptation of tissues by increasing oxygen extraction ratio ($O_2ER$).
  - Increase in $O_2ER$ helps in maintaining aerobic metabolism even with a decrease in oxygen delivery ($DO_2$) and/or an increase in metabolic demand of the tissues.
- At critical $DO_2$ ($cDO_2$) maximal $O_2ER$ is reached and any further decrease in $DO_2$ leads to tissue hypoxia and promotes anaerobic metabolism (or SHOCK STATE). Anaerobic metabolism in the tissue is reflected by increased production of lactate and a rise in serum lactate level (As seen in Fig. 11.1).
- Septic shock is characterized by abnormalities of macrocirculatory parameters (low cardiac output, low arterial pressure), microcirculation (microvascular abnormalities, endothelial dysfunction, capillary leak) and cellular metabolism (mitochondrial dysfunction and impaired oxygen utilization).
  - In the early stages of septic shock, profound vasodilation leads to a relative loss of stressed volume in the venous side, decreasing the venous return and cardiac output.
  - Additionally, patients with septic shock can have true hypovolemia, directly due to underlying source of infection, e.g. gastrointestinal volume loss resulting from ongoing diarrheal illness.
  - Vasodilatation also results in a fall in arterial blood pressure.
  - Certain subset of patients with septic shock can also develop poor cardiac contractility (also known as **Septic Cardiomyopathy**) that can contribute to tissue hypoperfusion.
  - In the later stages of septic shock (especially with delay in resuscitation) microcirculatory and cellular abnormalities predominate, with no further response to

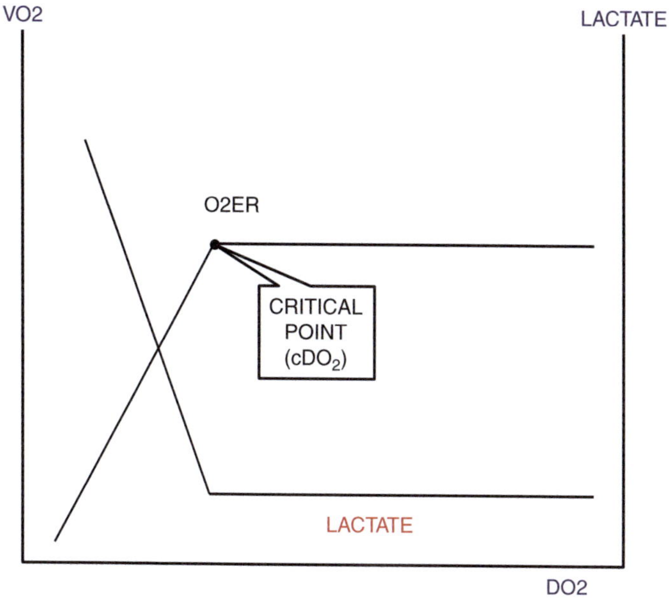


FIGURE 11.1 Schematic diagram showing the relationship between oxygen delivery and extraction. Critical point and anaerobic production of lactate. $DO_2$ oxygen delivered, $VO_2$ oxygen extracted, $O_2ER$ oxygen extraction ratio

increased flow from augmentation of cardiac output and/or arterial pressure. This later condition is described as "loss of coherence" between macro- and micro-hemodynamics. At this stage, any attempt to augment macro-hemodynamic parameters further can actually impair tissue perfusion further [4].

## 11.3 Recognition of Septic Shock

- Initial evaluation of the patient should focus on both recognition of septic shock (so that prompt resuscitative measures can be initiated) and identification of the possible site of infection (for early administration of appropriate antibiotic and control of source).

- A good history is the key to achieving both goals. History should be taken for any change (even trivial) in sensorium (especially in elderly patients) or any decrease in urine output over a period of several hours.
- Focus should also be on any systemic symptoms (e.g. throat pain, cough, pleuritic pain, gastrointestinal symptoms, dysuria, urgency, headache, seizure, etc.), travel history, exposure to possibly contaminated food or environment, insect or animal bite and any history of similar illness in the family.
- Bedside clinical examination should include evaluation for peripheral skin perfusion including skin temperature, skin rashes (Fig. 11.2), mottling or capillary refill

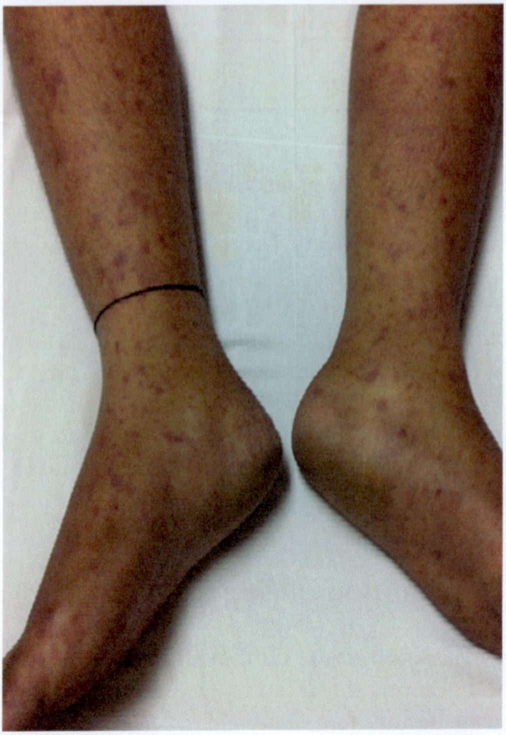

FIGURE 11.2 Young girl, presenting in shock state with typical rash of meningococcaemia

time, any evidence of bleeding from natural orifices and focused systemic examination (based on history).

- Blood and other appropriate body fluids should be sent for culture. This helps in identifying organisms responsible for infection and for streamlining antimicrobial therapy.
- Focused radiological investigations are necessary for identifying the source of infection and for planning appropriate source control.
- **Mottling:** Patchy discolouration of the skin or mottling, initially observed over the kneecap, is a specific indicator of poor skin perfusion. However, it may not be evident in dark-skinned individuals. Ait-Oufella and colleagues described a scoring system for skin mottling with higher score post initial resuscitation, predicting higher risk of mortality [5].
  - **Score 0:** No mottling.
  - **Score 1:** Coin size mottling localized to the centre of kneecap.
  - **Score 2:** Moderate mottling with area not exceeding the superior edge of the kneecap.
  - **Score 3:** Mottled area extending up to mid-thigh (Fig. 11.3).
  - **Score 4:** Mottling area up to the fold of the groin.
  - **Score 5:** Extremely severe. Area of mottling extending beyond the fold of the groin often in the whole-body surface (Fig. 11.4).
- **Capillary Refill Time:** Capillary refill time or CRT can be defined as the time required for the skin colour to return to baseline after application of blenching pressure at the nail bed or over the sternum. It is a sensitive indicator of blood flow in the distal capillary [6].
  - Repeated measurement of CRT is useful for follow-up of resuscitation adequacy and also for prognostication. ANDROMEDA-SHOCK investigators have described a simple and standardized method for bedside measurement of CRT (Fig. 11.5) [7].

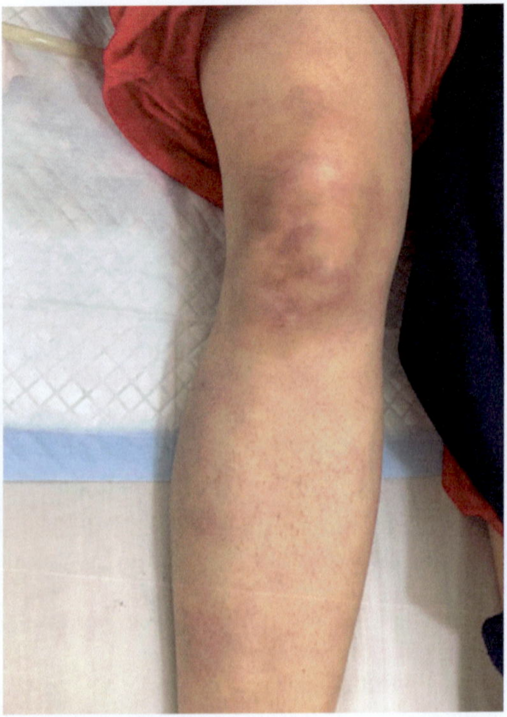

FIGURE 11.3 Middle-aged lady presenting with septic shock (urosepsis) with Stage 3 mottling

- With a glass slide apply firm pressure to the ventral surface of the distal phalanx of right index finger. Apply pressure until the skin goes blenched completely. Maintain this pressure for 10 seconds.
- Then release the pressure and measure the time (with a chronometer) taken for the return of normal skin colour.
- CRT of more than 3 seconds is considered abnormal.
- Value of CRT may be limited in patients with profound vasospasm, peripheral vascular disease, connective tissue disorders like scleroderma or in patients with very dark skin.

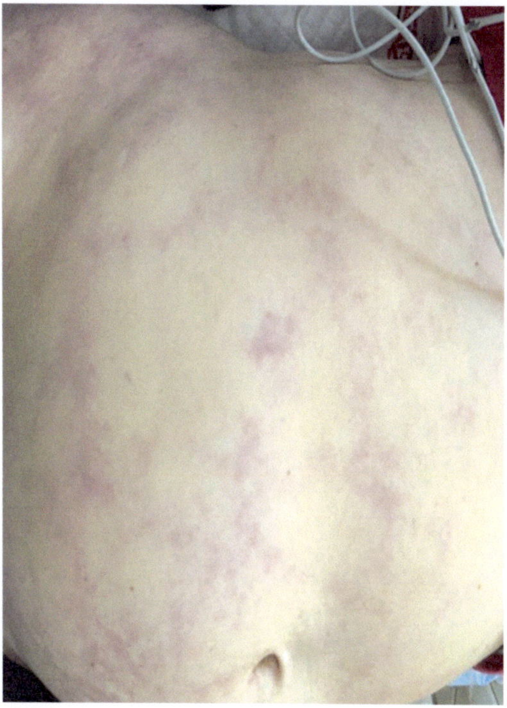

Figure 11.4 Stage 5 mottling in a middle-aged cirrhotic man with septic shock

- **Blood Pressure:** As per the new definition, septic shock can be identified clinically as sepsis with persistent hypotension or requiring vasopressors to maintain mean arterial pressure of 65 mmHg and having a serum lactate level > 2 mmol/L, despite adequate fluid resuscitation [3].
  - Surviving sepsis guideline includes hypotension as an essential criterion for defining septic shock [8]. However, there are several limitations to this simple assumption.
  - Hypotension is defined variably from a systolic blood pressure of below 100 or 90 mmHg or a mean arterial pressure below 65 mmHg.

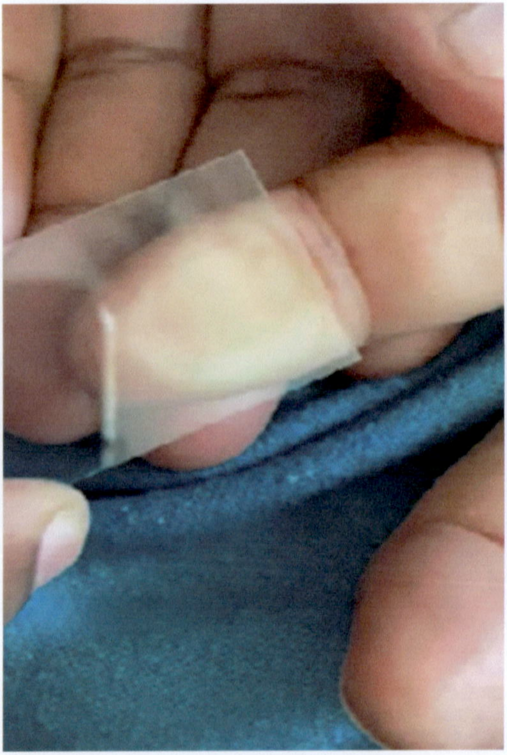

FIGURE 11.5 Testing for capillary refill time. (As proposed by ANDROMEDA-SHOCK Trial Investigators)

- In chronically hypertensive patients any lowering of blood pressure from their baseline value may be perceived by the body as detrimental and the baseline value may not be known at presentation.
- All hypotension may not be associated with poor organ perfusion.
- Hypotension may be a delayed presentation in some patients because of compensatory response. In fact, high lactate values without hypotension in patients with septic shock (so-called **"CRYPTIC SHOCK"**) have similar bad prognosis as overt shock with hypotension [9].

- **Lactate:** In hypoperfusion state, anaerobic glycolysis promotes increased production of pyruvate, which in turn is converted to lactate resulting in hyperlactatemia. In physiological state pyruvate mostly enters the Krebs' cycle for further aerobic metabolism.
  - German physician Johann Joseph Scherer is credited with the first description of an association between high lactate and severity of illness [10]. High value of serum lactate is associated with poor prognosis in patients with sepsis [3].
  - Surviving sepsis guideline suggests repeated measurement of Lactate during resuscitation process of septic shock [8]. However, measurement of lactate for diagnosis and follow-up in shock states have some limitations.
  - Lactate value may not be elevated in every patient in shock. However, absence of hyperlactatemia indicates better prognosis in these patients [9].
  - Stress-related adrenergic hyperactivity may be associated with hyperglycaemia, increased glycolysis and increased pyruvate production. This may lead to high production of lactate.
  - Lactate is metabolized in the liver by Cori cycle and impaired hepatic function may decrease the clearance of lactate.
  - Mitochondrial dysfunction may limit pyruvate metabolism.
  - Lactate clearance may be impaired by relative and absolute deficiency of thiamine, a co-factor required for the metabolism of lactate.
  - Many medications, e.g. metformin, anti-retroviral drugs are associated with lactic acidosis.
  - Lactate is a widely available laboratory parameter in big hospitals, as most commercially available blood gas machine gives lactate value in their printed report. But the availability of lactate value may be an issue in resource-limited setting.
  - Despite its several limitations, all hyperlactatemia must be investigated further. A differentiation must be established promptly between "Hypoperfusion related" and

"non-hypoperfusion related" cause of lactate elevation, so that an early and appropriate management can be initiated [9]. At the bedside, simple measurement of CRT, central venous oxygen saturation ($S_{cv}O_2$) and veno-arterial partial pressure of carbon dioxide difference ($P_{v-a}CO_2$) can easily differentiate between these two [10].

- **SvO2/ScvO2:** Oxygen saturation measured from the mixed venous sample (mixed venous oxygen saturation, $S_vO_2$), obtained by insertion of Pulmonary Artery catheter.
  - $S_vO_2$ is used as a surrogate of oxygen delivery to the tissue and can indirectly reflect tissue perfusion.
  - $S_{cv}O_2$ or oxygen saturation of blood samples obtained from central venous catheter can be utilized as a surrogate of $S_vO_2$.
  - $S_vO_2 > 65\%$ or $S_{cv}O_2 > 70\%$ have been advocated by surviving sepsis campaign as one of the targets for resuscitation [8].
- **Bedside Ultrasound:** A useful way to quickly identify mechanisms of shock is a focused ultrasound performed at the bedside by a trained acute care physician [11]. In an appropriate clinical context ultrasound examination can help in three different ways:
  - In ruling out other causes of shock: Number of protocols (e.g. RUSH, FALLS, etc.) had been described for this purpose.
  - In identifying source of possible infection: Example consolidation pattern in lung ultrasound for pneumonia or fluid collection in pleural/peritoneal/pericardial cavity, localized abscess in liver or hydronephrosis of kidney.
  - In choosing correct resuscitation measure: No significant respirophasic variation in inferior caval diameter in a ventilated patient receiving at least 8 ml/Kg of tidal volume with no spontaneous breathing effort can help in taking a decision not to infuse further fluid.
- **Invasive Monitoring:** Evaluation of haemodynamic variables with placement of a pulmonary artery (PA) catheter

can help in differentiating between different types of shock.

- But with the availability of non-invasive diagnostic and monitoring techniques, PA catheter is no longer being used routinely in modern-day intensive care units.
- Moreover, PA catheter had fallen out of favour among acute care physicians because of some studies questioning the safety of PA catheter and others not showing any benefit of PA catheter in the early management of shock [12, 13].
- However, certain parameters obtained during invasive monitoring are still useful during the process of septic shock management.

- Figure 11.6 below gives an approach to septic shock diagnosis at the bedside.

## 11.4 Management of Septic Shock

- Management of septic shock is based on four main principles ["**E-R-O-S**" Principle as shown in Fig. 11.7]:
  - **E**arly recognition of shock state and identification of source of infection.
  - Rapid establishment of tissue **R**e-perfusion.
  - Providing support to failing **O**rgans.
  - Most importantly control of **S**ource of the problem by appropriate management of infection.
- In subsequent paragraphs, we shall be discussing the principles of intravenous fluid management in septic shock aiming to restore tissue perfusion rapidly.

### *11.4.1 Which Fluid?*

- There is now consensus in favour of using isotonic crystalloids as the initial fluid of choice in septic shock. This strategy is also supported by SSC guidelines [8].

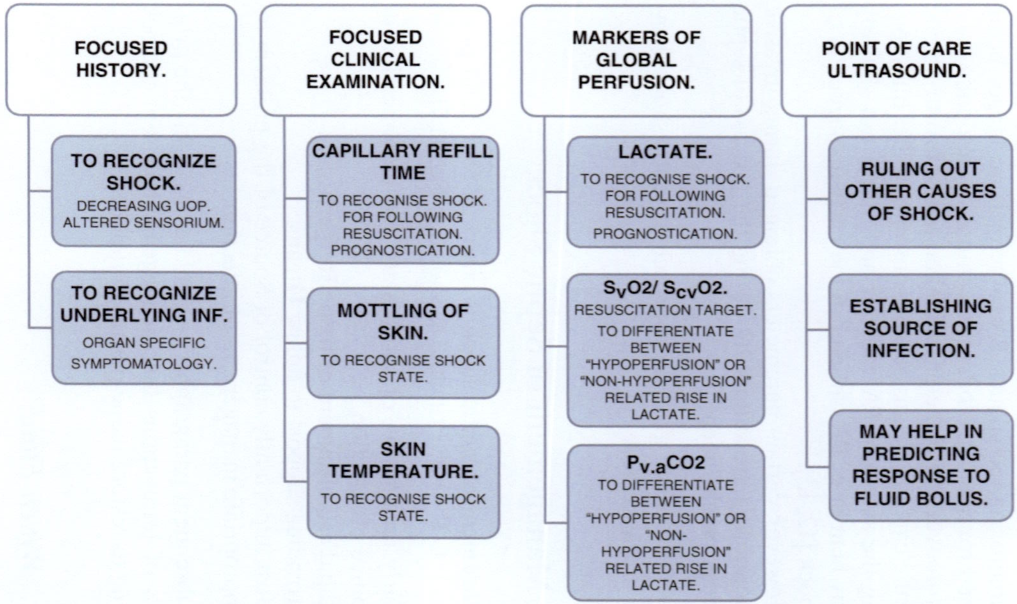


Figure 11.6 A holistic approach to the diagnosis of SEPTIC SHOCK. $S_vO_2$ mixed venous oxygen saturation, $S_{cv}O_2$ central venous oxygen saturation, $P_{v\text{-}a}CO_2$ veno-arterial carbon dioxide pressure difference

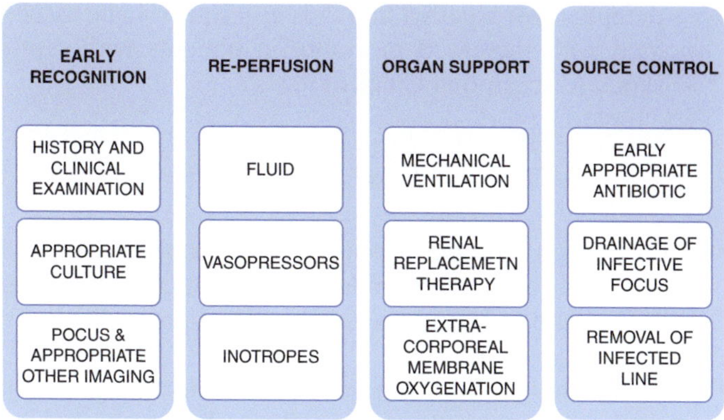


FIGURE 11.7 Four-Pillars of septic shock management (E-R-O-S)

- Hypotonic fluids should not be used for the purpose of resuscitation.
- Clinical and experimental studies have shown 0.9% Saline resuscitation to be associated with hyperchloremic metabolic acidosis with a potential for worse renal outcome and possible increase in mortality. Hence, 0.9% Saline should preferably be avoided during septic shock resuscitation unless other options are not available (discussed in Chap. 5).
- Balanced crystalloids are preferred crystalloid of choice. Several observational and randomized trials have confirmed relatively lesser renal dysfunction associated with balanced fluid resuscitation (discussed in Chap. 5). However, there is no clear advantage of any particular balanced fluid over others.

- Amongst colloids, only albumin infusion is found to be safe in patients with septic shock but its widespread use is limited by cost and availability.
  - Hyperoncotic albumin may be considered to reduce overall resuscitation volume (discussed in Chap. 6).
  - Synthetic colloids should not be used during septic shock resuscitation, as they have clearly been shown to be associated with worse renal outcomes and coagulation

defects. Hydroxyethyl Starch is also shown to be associated with increased mortality in patients with septic shock (discussed in Chap. 6).

### *11.4.2 How Much Fluid?*

- Resuscitation volume should be just optimal as fluid requirement of a patient follows a "U" shaped curve with both too little fluid and too much of fluid producing harm (Fig. 11.8).
- Patient's fluid requirement depends on underlying clinical condition. For example, resuscitation volume required for a patient with duodenal perforation and secondary peritonitis with septic shock will not be the same as a

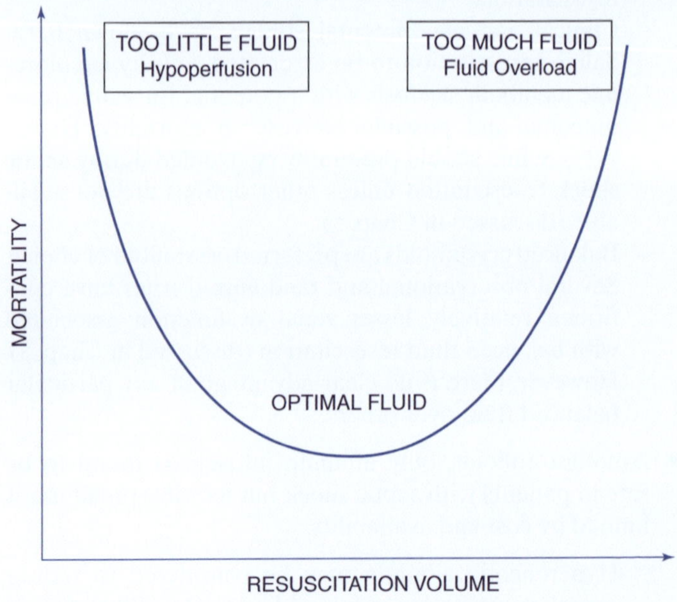


FIGURE 11.8 U-shaped curve showing harmful effect of both too much or too little fluid. Concept of optimal fluid at the bottom of the curve

hypoxemic patient on invasive ventilator with pneumonia and septic shock. Volume requirement also depends on the stage of resuscitation (as discussed in Chap. 10).

- **Rescue Phase:** Surviving Sepsis guideline suggests 30 ml/Kg of body weight as initial fluid bolus, to be started within 1 h of shock onset [8]. However, there is too little scientific evidence behind this recommendation.
  - More pragmatic approach should possibly be to follow Sir Thomas Latta's original description of fluid resuscitation way back in 1832, "…having no precedence to guide me I injected ounce after ounce of fluid closely observing the patient" [14].
  - Minimal fluid bolus to be administered at a time should be at least 4 ml/kg of body weight [15].
- **Optimization Phase:** After administration of initial fluid bolus during rescue phase of resuscitation further fluid boluses must be guided by appropriate tests for fluid responsiveness (discussed in Chap. 9). This strategy is also supported by SSC guidelines.
  - When tests for fluid responsiveness cannot be performed or they are not reliable, clinician should go ahead with a fluid challenge (discussed in Chap. 9).
  - Patient should be administered further fluid boluses only when he or she is in circulatory shock, is volume responsive (as judged by tests or fluid responsiveness or appropriately performed fluid challenge) and there is no obvious harm associated with further fluid boluses.
- **Stabilization Phase:** In this phase use of fluid boluses should be avoided, unless there is clear evidence of hypoperfusion and reasonable certainty about the benefit associated with boluses.
  - Maintenance fluids must be kept to the minimal.
- **Evacuation Phase:** Once the patient is adequately resuscitated and clinically stable, clinician should consider de-resuscitative measures in appropriately selected patients (as discussed in Chap. 10).

- **Restricted Fluid Strategy:** In every stage of resuscitation, maximal attempt should be made to keep the administered volume of fluid as minimal as possible. In the CLASSIC pilot study, a strategy restricting overall cumulative fluid balance was shown to have a trend towards better 90-day survival, lower ischemic events and statistically significant lower acute kidney injury events in patients with septic shock [16]. Several strategies can help in restricting fluid volumes in patients with septic shock and is discussed below.

  1. Norepinephrine by its venoconstriction effect can increase mean systemic filling pressure and in turn venous return (as discussed in Chaps. 1 and 8). Thus, early administration of Norepinephrine (after initial fluid bolus) is beneficial in reducing overall fluid resuscitation volume especially in patients with profound vasodilatation.

     – Profound vasodilatation in an individual patient can be identified by very low diastolic blood pressure (less than 40 mmHg).
     – Profound vasodilatation can also be recognized in the presence of a high diastolic shock index ≥2.3 [17]. Diastolic shock index is defined as the ratio between Heart Rate (in beats per minute) and Diastolic Blood Pressure (in mmHg)].
     – In "REFRESH" Study, a protocol utilizing early administration of norepinephrine after initial 1000 ml crystalloid bolus was found to restrict cumulative fluid balance at 6-h of resuscitation [18].

  2. Early administration of hyperoncotic albumin (20% or 25%) can potentially reduce overall fluid volume administered as seen in "SWIPE Study" data (discussed in Chap. 6) [19].
  3. To reduce overall cumulative fluid balance, clinician should keep an eye on "Fluid Creep" (defined as fluid administered during the administration of medications or flushing solutions) and avoid unnecessary prescription of maintenance fluid when patient can be fed via enteral route (discussed in Chap. 7) [20].

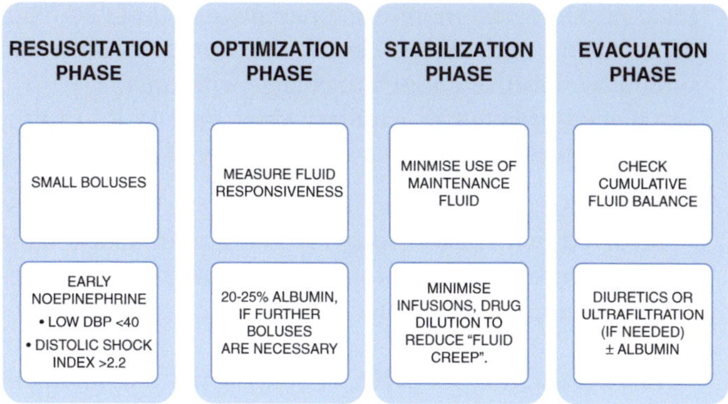


FIGURE 11.9 Suggested measures to reduce the cumulative fluid balance in different stages of resuscitation

- Figure 11.9 gives some suggested measures to reduce the cumulative fluid balance in different stages of fluid resuscitation ("ROSE" concept [21] is discussed in Chap. 9).

## *11.4.3 How (and What) to Monitor?*

- During the process of resuscitation patients should be monitored for improvement of physiological parameters including heart rate, mean arterial pressure, increase in urine output, improvement of peripheral perfusion parameters (especially capillary refill time), gradual normalization of central venous (or mixed venous) oxygen saturation and gradual improvement in lactate.
- Patients should also be monitored for any harmful consequences of resuscitation measures including fluid overload by continuous monitoring of oxygen saturation or appearance of B-Profile in lung ultrasound or increase in extravascular lung water and (in selected patients) measurement of intra-abdominal pressure.
- SSC guidelines suggest serial measurement of lactate to follow progress of resuscitation [8].

- Ideal physiological monitoring parameter should be readily available and cheap, can be measured reliably and should be sensitive enough to change with time.
- Serial measurement of capillary refill time (CRT) fulfils almost all these criteria in a vast majority of patients.
  - It is universally available (with no additional cost involved) with fastest recovery kinetics (of all available physiological parameters) and its normalization is associated with better regional perfusion and better prognosis [4].
  - In ANDROMEDA-SHOCK study serial measurement of CRT during septic shock resuscitation was shown to be correlated with better organ recovery compared to serial measurement of lactate (discussed in Box 11.1) [7].
  - Non-normalization of CRT in certain patients may suggest loss of hemodynamic coherence (and no benefit of additional macro-hemodynamic resuscitation).

**Box 11.1 "ANDROMEDA-SHOCK" Study [7]**

- **Research Question**: Is resuscitation guided by CRT associated with better clinical outcomes compared to Lactate-guided one?
- **Setting:** 28 Centres from 5 South American countries participated in the trial.
- **Patient:** 424 Septic shock patients resuscitated with step-by-step standardized resuscitation protocol were randomized to one of the two following groups.
- **Intervention:** Targeting normalization of CRT. CRT was measured every 30 min.
- **Control:** Targeting lactate normalization. Lactate was measured every 2 h (as lactate kinetics is relatively slow).
- **Outcome:** There was a trend towards better 28-day survival in CRT-guided group (34.9% vs 43.4%) but it was not statistically significant.

- There was a significant difference in organ dysfunction score (measured by SOFA) favouring CRT-guided group at 72-h.
- CRT-guided group received significantly lower resuscitation fluid at 8 h.
- There was no statistically significant difference between the two groups in ventilator-free days or RRT-free days or vasopressor-free days or ICU/Hospital Length of Stay.

### *11.4.4 What Should Be the End-Point of Resuscitation?*

- A holistic approach should be followed to decide end-point of resuscitation. Sometimes multiple parameters may be utilized to take a final call.
- In the landmark EGDT study by Emanuel Rivers and colleagues, aggressive resuscitation targeting multiple parameters (including $ScvO_2$) was shown to improve outcomes in patients with sepsis (as shown in Box 11.2) [22].

**Box 11.2 EGDT Study—Emanuel Rivers et al. [22]**

- **Research Question:** Is early goal-directed resuscitation of severe sepsis and septic shock patients in ED going to improve patient-centred outcomes compared to usual care?
- **Setting:** Emergency Department of a single large academic centre in the USA.
- **Patient:** 263 Patients admitted to ED with severe sepsis (i.e. Sepsis as per current definition) or Septic shock.
- **Intervention:** Aggressive resuscitation measures targeting $ScvO_2 > 70\%$ (measured continuously). CVP

Guided fluid, Blood Transfusion, Vasopressor and Dobutamine.

- **Control:** Usual care.
- **Outcome:** Intervention group received more fluid, less vasopressor. More inotropic support, more transfusion and by chance more appropriate antibiotics at 6-h.
  - However, at 72 h there is no difference in two groups in cumulative fluid volume received.
  - Significantly lower in-hospital (30.5% vs. 46.5%), 28-day (30.3% vs. 49.2%) and 60-day (44.3% vs. 55.6%) mortality was observed in the intervention group compared to control group).

- However, three more recent studies conducted across several continents could not confirm the results of Rivers' study (shown in Table 11.1) [23–25].
- Other resuscitation end-points could be normalization of CRT (as suggested in ANDROMEDA-SHOCK) or normalization of lactate (as suggested by Surviving Sepsis guideline).

## 11.5 Case Scenario (Continued)

- Mr. AA is in circulatory shock (altered sensorium, cool extremities, low blood pressure, high lactate), possibly septic shock (history of fever and clinical findings consistent with pneumonia).

TABLE 11.1 Summary of PROMISE, ARISE and PROMISE studies comparing Rivers' protocol with contemporary usual care in patients with septic shock

| | **PROCESS study [23]** | **ARISE study [24]** | **PROMISE study [25]** |
|---|---|---|---|
| Setting | 31 Centres. USA. | 51 Centres. Australia, NZ, Finland, Hongkong, Ireland. | 56 academic. UK. |
| Patient | Septic shock presented in ED. | Septic shock presented to ED. | Septic shock presented in ED. |
| No of patients | 1341. Randomized to 3 groups. | 1600. Randomized to 3 groups. | 1260. Randomized to 2 groups. |
| Intervention | – EGDT group: Rivers' protocol.<br>– Standard protocol group. | EGDT group: Rivers' protocol. | EGDT group: Rivers' protocol |
| Control | Usual care | Usual care | Usual care |
| Primary outcome | – No difference in 60-day mortality between groups. 21% vs. 18.2% vs. 18.9%. | – No difference in 90-day mortality between groups. 18.6% vs. 18.2%. | – No difference in 90-day mortality between groups. 29.5% vs. 29.2%. |

(continued)

TABLE 11.1 (continued)

| | **PROCESS study [23]** | **ARISE study [24]** | **PROMISE study [25]** |
|---|---|---|---|
| Secondary outcome | – Standard protocol group received group more fluid.<br>– Both protocol group received more vasopressors.<br>– EGDT group received more Dobutamine.<br>– No difference in 90-day mortality between groups. 31.9% vs. 30.8% vs. 33.7%.<br>– No difference in new-onset organ failure.<br>– No difference in duration of organ support. | – EGDT group received significantly more fluid, vasopressors, dobutamine and blood at 6-H.<br>– No difference in mortality at ICU or hospital discharge and at 28 days.<br>– Longer duration of stay at ED in EGDT group. But no difference in ICU or hospital LOS.<br>– No difference in MV/RRT utilization and duration. | – EGDT group received significantly more fluid, vasopressors, dobutamine and blood at 6-H.<br>– No difference in 28-day mortality.<br>– No difference in health-related quality of life or quality-adjusted life-year at 90 days.<br>– No difference in healthcare cost at 90 days. |

Table 11.1 (continued)

| | **PROCESS study [23]** | **ARISE study [24]** | **PROMISE study [25]** |
|---|---|---|---|
| Comments | – Rivers' trial was a proof-of-concept trial establishing firmly the need for early resuscitation in septic shock.<br>– Patient groups in Rivers' study and newer trials are not the same with gap of more than a decade between them.<br>– More patients in newer trials received early antibiotics and fluid bolus before enrolment.<br>– $ScvO_2$ at enrolment in Rivers' trial much lower suggesting enrolment of patients at an earlier stage of illness.<br>– Rivers' patients received ~13.5 L fluid at 72 h versus 6.5 L fluid in "PROMISE" showing a move towards "early aggressive" and "late restrictive" fluid therapy.<br>– Rivers' trial enrolled more chronic patients. | | |

- Bedside ultrasound performed by a trained clinician will be useful at this stage in establishing the diagnosis (consolidation pattern), ruling out other causes (pump function or possible cardiac tamponade) and for deciding the volume to be transfused.
- Apart from early administration of appropriate antibiotics, early aggressive resuscitation will be necessary to achieve a favourable outcome.
- In view of baseline hypoxemia, fluid administration needs to be cautious and every attempt should be made to restrict the cumulative volume of intravenous fluid.

**Take-Home Messages**

- Septic shock is a medical emergency and early recognition with focused history, clinical examination and basic laboratory tests is key to appropriate management with resuscitation, organ support and control of source.
- Goal of resuscitation is to establish tissue perfusion without causing undue harm due to the resuscitation process itself. Three key measures of resuscitation are intravenous fluid, administration of vasopressors and appropriate use of inotropic agents. A suggested approach to resuscitation of patients with septic shock is given in Fig. 11.10.
- Isotonic balanced crystalloids are first choice of intravenous fluid. Key is to administer small boluses of fluids and continuously monitoring improvement in hypoperfusion state.
- After initial fluid bolus, further administration of fluid should be guided by tests for fluid responsiveness (or fluid challenge).
- Early administration of vasopressors is useful in most patients for limiting cumulative fluid balance.
- A holistic approach should be followed to decide end-point of resuscitation.

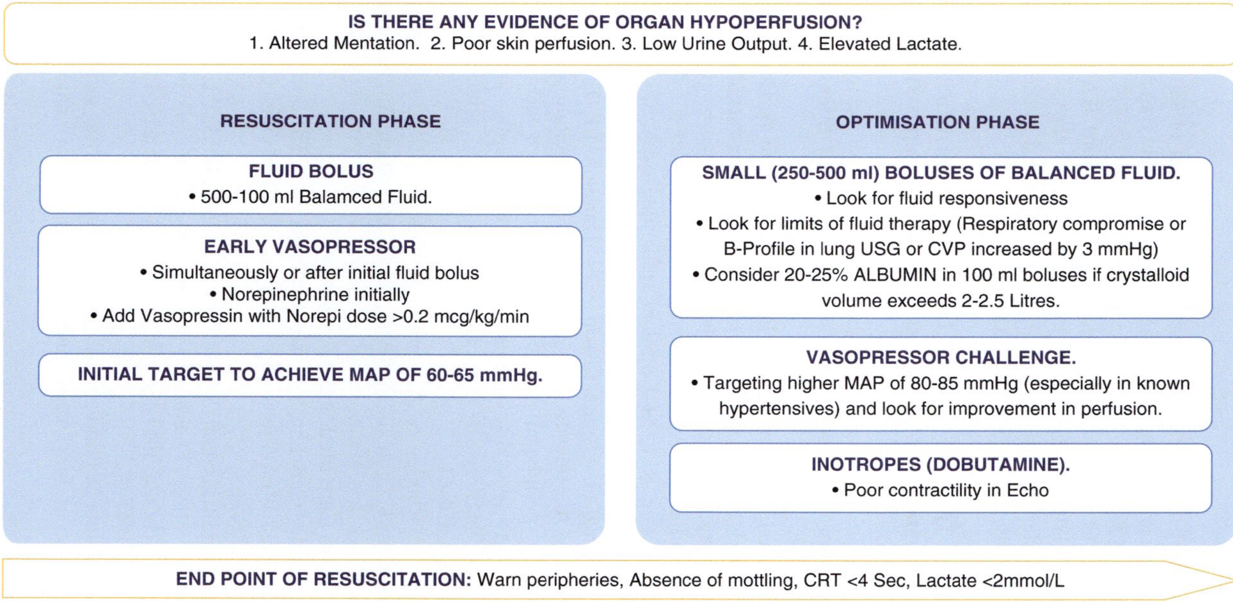


FIGURE 11.10 A suggested approach to resuscitation

## References

1. Weil MH, Shubin H. Proposed reclassification of shock states with special reference to distributive defects. Adv Exp Med Biol. 1971;23:13–23.
2. Rudd KE, Johnson SC, Agesa KM, Shackelford KA, Tsoi D, Kievlan DR, et al. Global, regional, and national sepsis incidence and mortality, 1990-2017: analysis for the global burden of disease study. Lancet. 2020;395:200–11.
3. Singer M, Deutschman CS, Seymour CW, Shankar-Hari M, Annane D, Bauer M, et al. The third international consensus definitions for sepsis and septic shock (sepsis-3). JAMA. 2016;315:801–10.
4. Hernández G, Teboul JL. Is the macrocirculation really dissociated from the microcirculation in septic shock? Intensive Care Med. 2016;42:1621–4.
5. Ait-Oufella H, Lemoinne S, Boelle PY, Galbois A, Baudel JL, Lemant J, et al. Mottling score predicts survival in septic shock. Intensive Care Med. 2011;37:801–7.
6. Ait-Oufella H, Bige N, Boelle PY, Pichereau C, Alves M, Bertinchamp R, et al. Capillary refill time exploration during septic shock. Intensive Care Med. 2004;40:958–64.
7. Hernández G, Ospina-Tascón GA, Damiani LP, Estenssoro E, Dubin A, Hurtado J, et al. Effect of a resuscitation strategy targeting peripheral perfusion status vs serum lactate levels on 28-day mortality among patients with septic shock: the ANDROMEDA-SHOCK randomized clinical trial. JAMA. 2019;321:654–64.
8. Evans L, Rhodes A, Alhazzani W, Antonelli M, Coopersmith CM, French C, et al. Surviving sepsis campaign: international guidelines for management of sepsis and septic shock 2021. Intensive Care Med. 2021;47:1181–247.
9. Hernandez G, Bruhn A, Castro R, Regueira T. The holistic view on perfusion monitoring in septic shock. Curr Opin Crit Care. 2012;18:280–6.
10. Kompanje EJ, Jansen TC, van der Hoven B, Bakker J. The first demonstration of lactic acid in human blood in shock by Johann Joseph Scherer (1814-1869) in January 1843. Intensive Care Med. 2007;33:1967–71.
11. Lichtenstein D. Fluid administration limited by lung sonography: the place of lung ultrasound in assessment of acute circula-

tory failure (the FALLS-protocol). Expert Rev Respir Med. 2012;6:155–62.
12. Connors AF Jr, Speroff T, Dawson NV, Thomas C, Harrell FE Jr, Wagner D, et al. The effectiveness of right heart catheterization in the initial care of critically ill patients. SUPPORT Investigators. JAMA. 1996;276:889–97.
13. Richard C, Warszawski J, Anguel N, Deye N, Combes A, Barnaud D, et al. Early use of the pulmonary artery catheter and outcomes in patients with shock and acute respiratory distress syndrome: a randomized controlled trial. JAMA. 2003;290:2713–20.
14. Latta T. Saline venous injection in cases of malignant cholera, performed while in the vapour-bath. Lancet. 1832;19(480):208–9.
15. Aya HD, Rhodes A, Chis Ster I, Fletcher N, Grounds RM, Cecconi M. Hemodynamic effect of different doses of fluids for a fluid challenge: a quasi-randomized controlled study. Crit Care Med. 2017;45:e161–8.
16. Hjortrup PB, Haase N, Bundgaard H, Thomsen SL, Winding R, Pettilä V, et al. Restricting volumes of resuscitation fluid in adults with septic shock after initial management: the CLASSIC randomised, parallel-group, multicentre feasibility trial. Intensive Care Med. 2016;42:1695–705.
17. Ospina-Tascón GA, Teboul JL, Hernandez G, Alvarez I, Sánchez-Ortiz AI, Calderón-Tapia LE, et al. Diastolic shock index and clinical outcomes in patients with septic shock. Ann Intensive Care. 2020;10(1):41.
18. Macdonald SPJ, Keijzers G, Taylor DM, Kinnear F, Arendts G, Fatovich DM, et al. Restricted fluid resuscitation in suspected sepsis associated hypotension (REFRESH): a pilot randomised controlled trial. Intensive Care Med. 2018;44:2070–8.
19. Mårtensson J, Bihari S, Bannard-Smith J, Glassford NJ, Lloyd-Donald P, Cioccari L, et al. Small volume resuscitation with 20% albumin in intensive care: physiological effects: the SWIPE randomised clinical trial. Intensive Care Med. 2018;44:1797–806.
20. van Regenmortel N, Verbrugghe W, Roelant E, Van den Wyngaert T, Jorens PG. Maintenance fluid therapy and fluid creep impose more significant fluid, sodium, and chloride burdens than resuscitation fluids in critically ill patients: a retrospective study in a tertiary mixed ICU population. Intensive Care Med. 2018;44:409–17.
21. Malbrain MLNG, Van Regenmortel N, Saugel B, De Tavernier B, Van Gaal PJ, Joannes-Boyau O, Teboul JL, et al. Principles of fluid management and stewardship in septic shock: it is time to

consider the four D's and the four phases of fluid therapy. Ann Intensive Care. 2018;8(1):66.
22. Rivers E, Nguyen B, Havstad S, Ressler J, Muzzin A, Knoblich B, Peterson E, Tomlanovich M, Early Goal-Directed Therapy Collaborative Group. Early goal-directed therapy in the treatment of severe sepsis and septic shock. N Engl J Med. 2001;345:1368–77.
23. Yealy DM, Kellum JA, Huang DT, Barnato AE, Weissfeld LA, Pike F, et al. A randomized trial of protocol-based care for early septic shock. N Engl J Med. 2014;370:1683–93.
24. Peake SL, Delaney A, Bailey M, Bellomo R, Cameron PA, Cooper DJ, et al. Goal-directed resuscitation for patients with early septic shock. N Engl J Med. 2014;371:1496–506.
25. Mouncey PR, Osborn TM, Power GS, Harrison DA, Sadique MZ, Grieve RD, et al. Trial of early, goal-directed resuscitation for septic shock. N Engl J Med. 2015;372:1301–11.

# Chapter 12
# Fluid Resuscitation in Haemorrhagic Shock

## 12.1 Case Scenario

Mr. RS, a 68-year-old male sustained multiple stab wounds in his abdomen by a knife while preventing a burglary attempt in his jewellery shop. He has been rushed to the emergency of the nearby hospital at 20–25 min distance from his shop. In the ED, he is conscious, obeying simple commands with a heart rate of 134/min and blood pressure of 50 mm Hg systolic on palpation. He is sweating profusely. Fresh blood is oozing from three wounds in his epigastric region and right upper quadrant of abdomen. After securing two large-bore intravenous line, ED physician decides to infuse 1 litre of warm Ringer's Lactate and initiate massive transfusion protocol.

### *12.1.1 What Are the Principles of Resuscitating Patients in Haemorrhagic Shock?*

Haemorrhagic shock is characterized by a lack of oxygen delivery to tissues due to profound blood loss. If not corrected in a timely fashion, haemorrhagic shock results in quick death. Major trauma is the single most important cause of haemorrhagic shock globally. Other causes include



S. Ghosh, *Handbook of Intravenous Fluids*,
https://doi.org/10.1007/978-981-19-0500-1_12

maternal haemorrhage (both antepartum and postpartum), gastrointestinal bleeding, perioperative bleeding or ruptured aneurysm. Annually an estimated 1.9 million people die from haemorrhagic shock worldwide; vast majority of these deaths are being from trauma. Rapid control of haemorrhage along with adequate and timely resuscitation are key factors in preventing mortality from haemorrhagic shock.

In this chapter, we shall discuss the pathophysiology of haemorrhagic shock and principles behind resuscitating such patients. Current evidence behind resuscitation of haemorrhagic shock is derived mostly from trauma research. Hence, our discussion will be centred mostly around bleeding trauma patients. Same principles can be extrapolated for resuscitation of other bleeding patients in haemorrhagic shock.

## 12.2 Pathophysiology

- Pathophysiology of haemorrhagic shock is quite complex. Multiple inter-related mechanisms involved are summarized below.
- Blood loss leads to depletion of red cells and haemoglobin, promoting anaerobic metabolism at cellular level. Anaerobic metabolism leads to accumulation of lactic acid, inorganic phosphates and oxygen-free radicals. With further depletion of ATP supply, cellular death finally ensues—through necrosis and apoptosis.
- Loss of blood volume activates the sympathoadrenal response as an immediate protective mechanism against hypovolemia. This leads to vasoconstriction in the non-vital organs, activation of neutrophils and other pro-inflammatory cells, ultimately resulting in increased endothelial permeability.
- Hypoperfusion and cellular injury lead to end-organ damage of liver, kidneys, skeletal muscles and later on of myocardium and brain producing multiple organ failure in survivors. Cellular and tissue damage also promote systemic inflammatory response syndrome and endothe-

lial damage. Endothelial damage further promotes shedding of glycocalyx and so-called endotheliopathy.

- Damage to blood vessels activates coagulation cascade locally and fibrinolysis at more distal organs (apparently to prevent microvascular thrombosis). However, excess fibrinolytic activity and auto-heparinization from glycocalyx shedding may lead to diffuse coagulopathy.
  - Thrombocytopenia resulting from the loss of whole blood and consumption of platelets during clotting process, along with platelet margination due to anaemia and reduced platelet activity due to multiple factors, further worsens the coagulopathy of trauma.
  - Iatrogenic factors can exacerbate coagulopathy. Overzealous crystalloid resuscitation can potentially dilute clotting factors concentration.
  - Crystalloid resuscitation can also indirectly worsen coagulopathy by promoting hypothermia (especially with cold fluid infusion) and by worsening acidosis (especially with large volume of 0.9% saline).
- Patients of haemorrhagic shock are at a high risk of hypothermia because of environmental exposure, resuscitation with cold resuscitation fluids, blood and blood products and depleted capacity of rewarming (due to lack of energy store).
  - Hypothermia leads to decreased function of the enzymes of coagulation cascade.
- Activities of the clotting factors are also severely impaired in the presence of acidosis.
  - Profound metabolic acidosis in turn is quite common in the presence of haemorrhagic shock both due to lactic acidosis induced by hypoperfusion state and because of large infusion of 0.9% Saline.
- The combination of coagulopathy, hypothermia and acidosis is also known as "**Lethal Triad**" and every effort should be made during trauma resuscitation to prevent and revert this lethal triad.

## 12.3 Initial Evaluation

- Initial evaluation should include both an assessment of approximate blood volume lost and identification of the source of bleeding. Looking for "hypotension" only to diagnose shock may mislead the clinician, because of robust compensatory mechanisms especially in young otherwise healthy individuals.
- **Classification of Hemorrhagic Shock** (Table 12.1): Advanced Trauma Life Support (ATLS) guideline has suggested the following classification scheme for assessing blood volume lost [1]. Unfortunately, ATLS classification tends to overestimate degree of tachycardia and underestimate mental status in assessing the volume loss [2].

Table 12.1 ATLS classification of haemorrhagic shock

| | **Class I** | **Class II** | **Class III** | **Class IV** |
|---|---|---|---|---|
| Blood loss (ml) | <750 | 750–1500 | 1500–2000 | >2000 |
| % Blood volume | 15% | 15%–30% | 30%–40% | >40% |
| Heart rate | Normal range | Normal to ↑ | ↑ | ↑↑ |
| Systolic pressure | Normal range | Normal range | Normal to ↓ | ↓ |
| Pulse pressure | Normal range | ↓ | ↓ | ↓ |
| Respiratory rate | Normal range | Normal range | Normal to ↑ | ↑ |
| Urine output | Normal range | Normal range | ↓ | ↓↓ |
| Sensorium | May be anxious | Anxious | Confused | Lethargic |

- **Shock Index**: Recent European guideline has recommended using "**Shock Index**" (SI) (defined as the ratio of heart rate and systolic blood pressure), to risk stratify bleeding trauma victims and to estimate the need for blood transfusion [3].
  - In a retrospective study, 2853 patients with trauma were classified into four groups based on SI at emergency admission—Group 1, SI <0.6, Group 2, SI ≥0.6 to <1, Group 3, SI ≥1 to <1.4 and Group 4, SI ≥1.4 [4].
  - Worsening of SI grade correlated well with injury severity score, need for blood transfusion and mortality.
  - Fifty-seven percent of group 4 patients required >10 units packed red blood cell (PRBC) transfusion before admission to ICU [4].
  - Overall mortality was as high as 39.8% in group 4 patients [4].
- In most patients, source of bleeding is obvious from history and physical examination. But it may not be so in a sizeable proportion of them.
  - Portable ultrasound machine is currently available in most emergency department and ICUs, as a bedside tool. Focused Assessment with Sonography for Trauma (FAST) examination has been suggested as the first-line modality to rapidly identify major intracavitary bleeding in chest, abdomen or pelvis especially in unstable patients [3]. Ultrasonography can also identify bleeding from abdominal aortic aneurysm or ruptured ectopic pregnancy.
  - However, the overall sensitivity of FAST examination is poor both in unstable and stable patients of traumatic haemorrhage [5].
- In hemodynamically stable patients of trauma with negative FAST especially in patients with high-impact injury should undergo a multislice (preferably whole-body) CT scan to identify missed source of haemorrhage [3].
  - Retroperitoneal space or thoracic aneurysms are sources of bleeding that is better evaluated with contrast-enhanced CT.

  - CT scanning should also be done in patients with positive FAST examination, provided they are hemodynamically stable, in order to identify additional injuries and to delineate the anatomy before taking the patient to Operating Room (OR) [3].

- Measurement of lactate and base excess is helpful for the assessment of global perfusion, for prognostication and for following up resuscitation.
- Haemoglobin and haematocrit should be measured at baseline and periodically. But transfusion of packed RBCs should not be based solely on haemoglobin/haematocrit value in an actively haemorrhaging patient.
- Measurement of coagulation parameters including platelet count, prothrombin time, partial thromboplastin time and fibrinogen level is useful in determining the need for plasma, platelet or cryoprecipitate transfusion following initial resuscitation.
  - Thromboelastography or rotational thromboelastometry, if available, may be useful to determine clot-formation kinetics and need for appropriate clotting factors replacement.
- Serial measurement of electrolytes especially sodium and potassium are a must during the process of resuscitation.
- Other useful laboratory parameters to be measured are kidney and liver function tests.

## 12.4 Management of Haemorrhagic Shock

- Two pillars of managing haemorrhagic shock include:
  A. Resuscitation aiming to maintain tissue perfusion with minimal or no damage due to resuscitation process itself ("**Damage Control Resuscitation**").
  B. "**Damage control surgery**" aiming to attain haemostasis rapidly either surgically, endoscopically or through angioembolization and to minimize contamination, keeping the definitive repair for a later period once the patient is stable.

- In subsequent paragraphs, we shall be focusing on "Damage Control Resuscitation" that in turn include the following key principles:
  - Restricted use of crystalloids
  - Haemostatic resuscitation
  - Prevention and treatment of hypothermia, coagulopathy and acidosis

## 12.5 Restricted Use of Crystalloids

- Overzealous resuscitation with crystalloids may be potentially harmful in patients with haemorrhagic shock, especially before the haemostasis is achieved.
  - Rise in blood pressure during rapid crystalloid boluses can potentially dislodge the newly formed clot plugging the bleeding point. This issue was recognized in the early twentieth century by WB Cannon, a US army surgeon, while he was caring for injured soldiers in World War 1 [6].
  - Large volume crystalloids can potentially increase the risk of bleeding by further worsening trauma-induced coagulopathy—dilutional coagulopathy and acidosis (discussed earlier in the chapter).
  - Synthetic colloids can worsen coagulopathy by themselves (discussed in Chap. 6).
  - Fluid overload can produce Global Increased Permeability Syndrome (GIPS), worsen hypoxemia, produce increased intra-abdominal pressure, increase intracranial pressure, increase pressure in limb compartment, further worsening morbidity and mortality.
- Three potential strategies can limit overall crystalloid infusion during trauma resuscitation (or in a larger context for haemorrhagic shock):
  1. Permissive hypotension
  2. Controlled resuscitation
  3. Delayed resuscitation

### *12.5.1 Permissive Hypotension*

- This is a strategy to resuscitate a patient of haemorrhagic shock to a blood pressure target lower than normal range, otherwise known as hypotensive resuscitation.
- This strategy is tested in two randomized trials in traumatic haemorrhagic shock, briefly shown in Table 12.2.
- Overall, permissive hypotension strategy is safe provided haemostasis is achieved early, but there is still no clarity on the permitted duration of hypotension.
  - In a murine haemorrhagic shock model, targeting a MAP of 50 to 60 mmHg was found to be safe and associated with less blood loss [9]. But if this permissive hypotension strategy is continued beyond 90-min, ani-

TABLE 12.2 Randomized studies evaluating effects of permissive hypotension in traumatic haemorrhagic shock

| | **Dutton et al [7]** | **Morrison et al [8]** |
|---|---|---|
| Setting | Single US Trauma Centre. RCT. | Single US Trauma Centre. RCT |
| Patients | Trauma patients presenting to study centre in Haemorrhagic shock. N = 110 | Traumatic haemorrhagic shock requiring emergency surgery. Randomized in the operating room. N = 90 |
| Intervention | • Fluid resuscitation targeting SBP 70 mmHg ("low") before achieving haemostasis. | • MAP permitted to go up to the lowest value of 50 mmHg before active resuscitation ["LMAP"]. |
| Control | • Fluid resuscitation targeting SBP >100 mmHg ("conventional") before achieving haemostasis. | • MAP permitted to go up to the lowest value of 65 mmHg before active resuscitation ["HMAP"]. |

Table 12.2 (continued)

| | **Dutton et al [7]** | **Morrison et al [8]** |
|---|---|---|
| Outcome | • Half the patients had penetrating trauma.<br>• Significant difference in SBP target between groups (114 vs 100 mmHg).<br>• Four deaths in each group.<br>• No difference in duration of active haemorrhage. | • Mostly patients had penetrating trauma (84/90).<br>• Actual MAP between groups not different (64.4 vs 68.5 mmHg).<br>• LMAP group received significantly lower intra-operative blood products and fluid.<br>• LMAP group had significantly lower likelihood of developing postoperative coagulopathy.<br>• Significantly lower immediate postoperative death (within 24-h) in LMAP group.<br>• Trend towards lower 30-day mortality in LMAP group. |

mals suffered irreversible organ dysfunction and significant increase in mortality [9].

- Although the target blood pressure could not be maintained in both studies (obviously because of body's physiological response), this strategy can potentially limit resuscitation volume, blood products, coagulopathy and can perhaps have a beneficial effect in terms of mortality.
  - However, this strategy cannot be applied in patients with associated traumatic brain injury, as maintaining cerebral perfusion pressure is essential to minimize secondary neuronal damage.

## *12.5.2 Controlled Resuscitation*

- Controlled resuscitation can be defined as a strategy to limit the volume of fluid to be administered especially in out-of-hospital setting.
- This strategy was tested in randomized "Resuscitation Outcome Consortium (ROC)" study (see Table 12.3). In

TABLE 12.3 Studies evaluating controlled resuscitation in traumatic haemorrhagic shock

| | **Brown et al. [10]** | **Schreiber et al. [11]** |
|---|---|---|
| Setting | Post-hoc, propensity-adjusted analysis of data originally collected for the proteomic and genomic response to blunt injury.<br>7 US Trauma centres. | Out of hospital setting. 19 emergency medical service (EMS) Systems from the USA.<br>Randomized control trial. |
| Patients | Blunt trauma patients transported from the scene who had record available for crystalloid received.<br>Injury severity scale >15.<br>N = 1216 | Trauma patients with pre-hospital hypotension (SBP <90 mmHg).<br>N = 192 |
| Intervention | Patients receiving LOW (<500 ml) crystalloid in pre-hospital. | Controlled resuscitation (CR). 250 ml of crystalloid if radial pulse not palpable or SBP <70 mmHg. Further 250 ml boluses to maintain radial pulse or SBP >70 mmHg. |
| Control | Patients receiving HIGH (>500 ml) crystalloid in pre-hospital. | Standard Resuscitation (SR). Initial 2000 ml crystalloid bolus and further boluses to maintain SBP >110 mmHg. |

TABLE 12.3 (continued)

| | Brown et al. [10] | Schreiber et al. [11] |
|---|---|---|
| Outcome | • In patients without pre-hospital hypotension (SBP >90 mmHg) HIGH crystalloid was associated with increased mortality and acute coagulopathy.<br>• In patients with pre-hospital hypotension SBP <90 mmHg) HIGH crystalloid was associated with improvement in pre-hospital systolic pressure on ED arrival (mean 104 mmHg).<br>• Each 1 mmHg increase in SBP in this subset of patients, improved the mortality by 2%. | • One-third of patients had penetrating trauma.<br>• Difference in average crystalloid volume administered was 1000 ml (1 litre in CR group and 2 litres in SR group).<br>• 24-h mortality was marginally higher in SR group (adjusted odds ratio 0.39 [95% CI: 0.12, 1.26]).<br>• 24-h mortality difference was significant only in blunt trauma; not in penetrating trauma.<br>• No difference in ICU-free days, ventilator-free days, renal injury and renal failure between groups. |

another study, Brown and colleagues performed a post-hoc analysis of data collected from a large multicentre cohort study and examined the effect of high or low volume resuscitation for trauma patients in pre-hospital setting (see Table 12.3).

- Based on the current evidence, crystalloids should be administered in pre-hospital setting only if the SBP is <70 mmHg. Crystalloid administration should be in small boluses (~250 ml of warm balanced fluids).
- But this above recommendation is not applicable in patients with associated traumatic brain injury and when there is significant delay in transporting the patient to a trauma centre or to nearest hospital [9].

## *12.5.3 Delayed Resuscitation*

- This is a strategy to delay the resuscitation altogether till some haemostasis is achieved.
- In a landmark study, Bickell and colleagues observed that delaying aggressive fluid resuscitation till operative intervention improves outcome in hypotensive patients with penetrating torso trauma [12] (see Box 12.1).

**Box 12.1 Bickell Study [12]**

- **Setting:** Single US trauma centre.
- **Patients:** Patients >16 years with penetrating injury to torso and recorded SBP <90 mmHg at the time of assessment by paramedics. N = 592.
- **Intervention:** Intravenous fluid resuscitation was delayed till operative intervention—both in pre-hospital and intra-hospital setting (Delayed Resuscitation Group).
- **Control:** Patients were resuscitated in the standard manner with rapid crystalloid infusion in pre-hospital setting, which was continued in the hospital with additional blood and blood products (Immediate Resuscitation Group).
- **Primary Outcome:** 8% increase in hospital survival in delayed resuscitation group (70% versus 62%).
- **Secondary Outcome:**
  - Delayed resuscitation group received significantly lower crystalloid in pre-hospital (92 ml vs 870 ml), in-hospital before Operation Theatre (283 ml vs 1608 ml) and lower packed RBC in-hospital before Operation Theatre (11 ml vs 133 ml).
  - Haemoglobin% was higher and prothrombin time was lower in delayed resuscitation group on ED arrival.
  - Hospital length of stay was longer in immediate resuscitation group.

- The impressive results of Bickell study have never been replicated in any other study or in patients with blunt trauma and haemorrhagic shock. However, no study till date has shown any harm associated with this strategy.

## 12.6 Which Fluid?

- There is now an impressive body of evidence supporting balanced crystalloids in vast majority of patients requiring fluid resuscitation, because of their low chloride content and higher SID resulting in less acidosis, compared to 0.9% Saline (discussed further in Chap. 5). Moreover, with higher sodium content, 0.9% Saline has higher propensity to produce tissue oedema.
  - However, in patients with associated traumatic brain injury, resuscitation fluids with higher osmolality should be preferred (0.9% Saline or Sterofundin) to reduce aggravation of cerebral oedema by hypotonic fluid infusion.
- With no study showing any clear benefit in the setting of haemorrhagic shock and some other studies showing potential harm associated with them, colloids cannot be recommended for resuscitation in patients with haemorrhagic shock (discussed further in Chap. 6).
- Hypertonic saline infusion is suggested by some experts in traumatic haemorrhagic shock patients especially in pre-hospital settings. Suggested rationales for hypertonic saline infusion are reduction in volume of resuscitation fluid and improvement of cerebral perfusion in patients with traumatic brain injury.
  - However, two large randomized trials by Resuscitation Outcome Consortium (ROC) in patients with traumatic brain injury [13] and in traumatic hypovolemic shock [14] were stopped prematurely as they did not show any benefit of hypertonic saline. In addition, both studies were associated with a potential for harm.

  - Based on the results of these two trials, hypertonic saline cannot be recommended in the setting of haemorrhagic shock.

- All fluids infused should be warm to match the normal body temperature to avoid hypothermia.

## 12.7 Haemostatic Resuscitation

- Central aspect of haemorrhagic shock pathophysiology is loss of haemoglobin (RBCs) along with blood volume, platelets and coagulation factors. Early replacement of haemoglobin is essential to maintain oxygen delivery to the tissue.
- Replacement of only haemoglobin and blood volume can deplete already depleted coagulation factors and platelet further. Hence, the concept of **Haemostatic Resuscitation** is developed that caters for early replacement of haemoglobin (RBCs) as well as blood volume, fresh frozen plasma (FFP) and platelets.
  - The concept of haemostatic resuscitation was established firmly after the 2007 landmark publication by Borgman and colleagues [15].
  - It was a retrospective analysis of 246 traumatic haemorrhagic shock patients admitted to the combat support hospital in Iraq, who had received massive transfusion, i.e. ≥10 units of packed red blood cell (PRBC).
  - Median injury severity scale was 18 for all patients with an overall mortality of 28%.
  - High ratio of plasma to PRBC was independently associated with survival, primarily by decreasing early (<4 h from admission) death due to haemorrhage.
  - A ratio 1:1.4 ("High Ratio") had the best chance of survival compared to a ratio 1:2.5 ("Medium Ratio) and 1:8 ("Low Ratio"). Overall mortality rates were 65%, 34% and 19% for low, medium and high ratio groups with corresponding haemorrhagic mortality rates of 92.5%, 78% and 37% [15].

- Patients with haemorrhagic shock require early transfusion of substantial amount of blood and blood products to maintain both tissue perfusion and haemostasis. Massive transfusion is arbitrarily defined as the transfusion of at least 10 units of PRBC over 24 h period [16].
  - It is important to identify early, patients who may require massive transfusion in order to facilitate transfusion of PRBCs, FFPs and Platelets in a balanced ratio as quickly as possible (so-called Massive Transfusion Protocol [MTP]).
  - The following criteria may be used to trigger MTP activation (originally developed for trauma but may be useful in other scenarios too) [16].
    1. ABC Score 2 or more. [ABC or Assessment of Blood Consumption score was developed to predict need for Massive Transfusion in Trauma with each of the following criteria carrying 1-point: 1. Penetrating Mechanism, 2. Systolic Blood Pressure (SBP) in Emergency Department (ED) <90 mmHg, 3. Heart Rate in ED >120/min and 4. Positive FAST Examination).
    2. Persistent hemodynamic instability
    3. Active bleeding requiring surgical or other intervention
    4. Blood transfusion requiring early in the trauma bay or emergency department

- One of the major criticisms of Borgman study was a possibility of "Survival Bias". That means those patients who survived long enough only received FFP (as thawing of FFP typically takes 30–40 min).
  - To overcome this bias, Holcomb and colleagues performed a multicentre observational study where they included trauma patients who survived first 30 min after admission and who had received at least one unit of PRBC within 6 h of admission and at least 3 units of blood products within 24 h [17]. Findings from this study further substantiated the association between higher plasma and platelet with decreased mortality during the first 24 h.

  - Interestingly, the study did not find any association between mortality and plasma/platelet ratio in patients who survived initial 24 h [17].

- Ratio of FFP: Platelet: PRBC more than 1:1:1 was found to achieve better haemostasis and fewer death due to exsanguination at 24-h in a randomized control study. But a ratio higher than this did not result in an additional improvement in mortality both at 24 h and at 30 days [18].

## 12.8 Other Measures

- **Achieving Haemostasis:** As discussed at the beginning of this chapter, the single most important measure to improve survival in patients with haemorrhagic shock is the early control of bleeding surgically or endoscopically or by angioembolization. Further discussion on the subject is beyond the scope of this book.
- **Anti-fibrinolytic agents:** Early administration (within 8-h) of tranexamic acid had shown to safely reduce mortality in bleeding trauma patients compared to placebo in the large multicentre CRUSH-2 trial [19]. Tranexamic acid dose used in CRUSH-2 was 1 g as intravenous bolus over 10 min followed by an infusion of 1 g over 8 h and should be used for all patients in haemorrhagic shock unless absolutely contraindicated.
- **Reversal of Anticoagulation:** In bleeding patients on therapeutic anticoagulation, must receive appropriate measures for reversal of anticoagulation either by specific anti-dote (e.g. Vitamin K for warfarin or Idarucizumab for Dabigatran) or appropriate replacement of clotting factors (FFPs or three/four factors Prothrombin Complex Concentrate for Warfarin or oral factor Xa inhibitors) or haemodialysis to remove anticoagulants from circulation (e.g. dabigatran).
- **Recombinant factor VIIa:** As an adjunct to usual therapy, it has been shown to reduce blood products use especially

in blunt trauma patients [20]. Recombinant factor VIIa has also been used in other desperate scenarios like post-partum haemorrhage [21]. But its use must also be balanced against cost and potential risk of thrombosis.

- **Correction of coagulopathy** is a priority with appropriate usage of platelet (preferably single donor or if not, with random donor), fresh frozen plasma and cryoprecipitate.
- **Hypothermia Correction:** Hypothermia must be avoided and corrected early by active rewarming. All fluids and blood products should be pre-warmed to body temperature before transfusion.
- **Prevention of Acidosis:** All measures must be taken to prevent worsening acidosis.
- **Vasopressors:** In life-threatening hypotension, vasopressors especially norepinephrine must be started immediately (as discussed in Chap. 8).
- **Blood Transfusion:** Haemoglobin and haematocrit must be monitored frequently even after haemostasis is achieved. In trauma situations suggested target haemoglobin should be between 7 and 9 g/dl [3]. Similarly in upper GI bleeding, a transfusion strategy with a haemoglobin level of 7 g/dl as a trigger for blood transfusion is found to be safe [22]. Similarly, in obstetric haemorrhage haemoglobin level of 7 g/dl has been suggested as transfusion trigger [23].
- **Calcium:** Calcium must be supplemented appropriately, especially after massive transfusion.

## 12.9 Case Scenario (Continued)

- Mr. RS is in haemorrhagic shock following penetrating abdominal trauma. Considering, systolic blood pressure as low as 50 mmHg, resuscitation must be initiated immediately with 500 ml of warm lactated Ringer solution with perhaps simultaneous initiation of norepinephrine infusion. Immediate target blood pressure should be SBP of at least 70 mmHg.

- Massive transfusion protocol must be initiated and as early as possible blood products must be transfused with FFP: Platelet: PRBC at a ratio of 1:1:1.
- FAST evaluation should be done in the emergency department.
- Surgical team must be alerted so that the patient can be taken up for OR to achieve early haemostasis. Need for pre-operative contrast-enhanced CT scan to delineate anatomy better should be at the discretion of the operating team and the decision should be taken based on the patient's hemodynamic stability following early resuscitation.
- Post-haemostasis, patient should be managed in the ICU where further resuscitation should be continued targeting tissue perfusion, support should be provided to dysfunctional organs and triad of hypothermia, coagulopathy and acidosis must be corrected.
- If necessary, the patient should be taken up for definitive surgery once he is stable after 3–4 days.

**Take-Home Messages**

- Cornerstone of managing haemorrhagic shock is early achievement of haemostasis.
- Resuscitation measures should focus on early initiation of blood products transfusion or haemostatic resuscitation, restricted crystalloid infusion and taking all steps to prevent and correct hypothermia, coagulopathy and acidosis.
- A suggested algorithm for managing haemorrhagic shock in different settings is given in Fig. 12.1. Aim should be to minimize duration of stay in every setting as much as possible based on local resources and expertise.

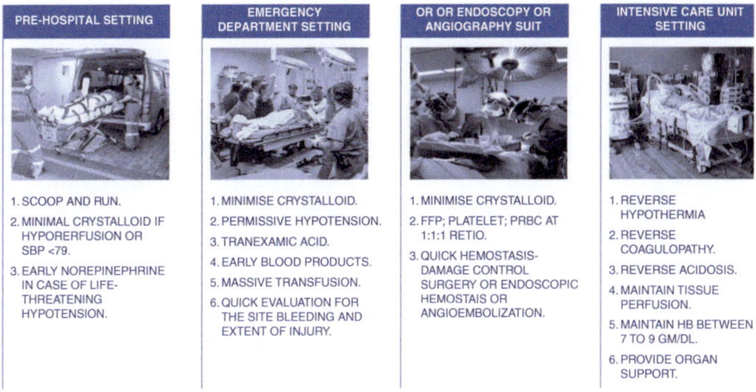


FIGURE 12.1 Suggested algorithm for managing haemorrhagic shock

## References


1. American College of Surgeons Committee on Trauma. ATLS® student manual 10th edition. Chicago: American College of Surgeons; 2018.
2. Mutschler M, Nienaber U, Brockamp T, Wafaisade A, Wyen H, Peiniger S, et al. A critical reappraisal of the ATLS classification of hypovolemic shock: does it really reflect clinical reality? Resuscitation. 2013;84:309–13.
3. Spahn DR, Bouillon B, Cerny V, Duranteau J, Filipescu D, Hunt BJ, et al. The European guideline on management of major bleeding and coagulopathy following trauma: fifth edition. Crit Care. 2019;23:R98.
4. Mutschler M, Nienaber U, Brockamp T, Wafaisade A, Fabian T, Paffrath T, Bouillon B, Maegele M, Trauma Register DGU. Renaissance of base deficit for the initial assessment of trauma patients: a base deficit-based classification for hypovolemic shock developed on data from 16,305 patients derived from the Trauma Register DGU(R). Crit Care. 2013;17:R42.
5. Carter JW, Falco MH, Chopko MS, Flynn WJ Jr, Wiles Iii CE, Guo WA. Do we really rely on fast for decision-making in the management of blunt abdominal trauma? Injury. 2015;46:817–21.
6. Cannon WB, Fraser J, Cowell EB. The preventive treatment of wound shock. JAMA. 1918;70:618–21.

7. Dutton RP, Mackenzie CF, Scalea TM. Hypotensive resuscitation during active hemorrhage: impact on in-hospital mortality. J Trauma. 2002;52:1141–6.
8. Morrison CA, Carrick MM, Norman MA, Scott BG, Welsh FJ, Tsai P, et al. Hypotensive resuscitation strategy reduces transfusion requirements and severe postoperative coagulopathy in trauma patients with hemorrhagic shock: preliminary results of a randomized controlled trial. J Trauma. 2011;70:652–63.
9. Li T, Zhu Y, Hu Y, Li L, Diao Y, Tang J, Liu L. Ideal permissive hypotension to resuscitate uncontrolled hemorrhagic shock and the tolerance time in rats. Anesthesiology. 2011;114:111–9.
10. Brown JB, Cohen MJ, Minei JP, Maier RV, West MA, Billiar TR, et al. Goal-directed resuscitation in the prehospital setting: a propensity-adjusted analysis. J Trauma Acute Care Surg. 2013;74:1207–12.
11. Schreiber MA, Meier EN, Tisherman SA, Kerby JD, Newgard CD, Brasel K, et al. A controlled resuscitation strategy is feasible and safe in hypotensive trauma patients: results of a prospective randomized pilot trial. J Trauma Acute Care Surg. 2015;78:687–95.
12. Bickell WH, Wall MJ Jr, Pepe PE, Martin RR, Ginger VF, Allen MK, Mattox KL. Immediate versus delayed fluid resuscitation for hypotensive patients with penetrating torso injuries. N Engl J Med. 1994;331:1105–9.
13. Bulger EM, May S, Brasel KJ, Schreiber M, Kerby JD, Tisherman SA, et al. Out-of-hospital hypertonic resuscitation following severe traumatic brain injury: a randomized controlled trial. JAMA. 2010;304:1455–64.
14. Bulger EM, May S, Kerby JD, Emerson S, Stiell IG, Schreiber MA, et al. Out-of-hospital hypertonic resuscitation after traumatic hypovolemic shock: a randomized, placebo-controlled trial. Ann Surg. 2011;253:431–41.
15. Borgman MA, Spinella PC, Perkins JG, Grathwohl KW, Repine T, Beekley AC, et al. The ratio of blood products transfused affects mortality in patients receiving massive transfusions at a combat support hospital. J Trauma. 2007;63:805–13.
16. Chang R, Holcomb JB. Optimal fluid therapy for traumatic hemorrhagic shock. Crit Care Clin. 2017;33:15–36.
17. Holcomb JB, del Junco DJ, Fox EE, Wade CE, Cohen MJ, Schreiber MA, et al. The prospective, observational, multicenter, major trauma transfusion (PROMMTT) study: comparative

effectiveness of a time-varying treatment with competing risks. JAMA Surg. 2013;148:127–36.
18. Holcomb JB, Tilley BC, Baraniuk S, Fox EE, Wade CE, Podbielski JM, et al. Transfusion of plasma, platelets, and red blood cells in a 1:1:1 vs a 1:1:2 ratio and mortality in patients with severe trauma: the PROPPR randomized clinical trial. JAMA. 2015;313:471–82.
19. Shakur H, Roberts I, Bautista R, Caballero J, Coats T, Dewan Y, et al. Effects of tranexamic acid on death, vascular occlusive events, and blood transfusion in trauma patients with significant haemorrhage (CRASH-2): a randomised, placebo-controlled trial. Lancet. 2010;376:23–32.
20. Boffard KD, Riou B, Warren B, Choong PI, Rizoli S, Rossaint R, Axelsen M, Kluger Y, NovoSeven Trauma Study Group. Recombinant factor VIIa as adjunctive therapy for bleeding control in severely injured trauma patients: two parallel randomized, placebo-controlled, double-blind clinical trials. J Trauma. 2005;59:8–15.
21. Ahonen J, Jokela R. Recombinant factor VIIa for life-threatening post-partum haemorrhage. Br J Anaesth. 2005;94:592–5.
22. Villanueva C, Colomo A, Bosch A, Concepción M, Hernandez-Gea V, Aracil C, et al. Transfusion strategies for acute upper gastrointestinal bleeding. N Engl J Med. 2013;368:11–21.
23. Muñoz M, Stensballe J, Ducloy-Bouthors AS, Bonnet MP, De Robertis E, Fornet I, et al. Patient blood management in obstetrics: prevention and treatment of postpartum haemorrhage. A NATA consensus statement. Blood Transfus. 2019;17:112–36.

# Chapter 13
# Fluid Management in Diarrhoeal Diseases

## 13.1 Case Scenario

Mr. MS, a 54-year-old otherwise healthy male is admitted to the emergency department with history of frequent passage of watery stool for the past 12 h. He is also having repeated episodes of vomiting. Stool contains no blood or mucous. There is no fever or pain in abdomen. Family gives history of him returning home a night before after a 7-days official visit to coastal areas of Bengal and Odisha. On examination, he seems to be lethargic with dry tongue, evidence of loss of skin turgor with feeble radial pulse 128/min, rapid shallow breathing. Capillary refill time is more than 10 s. No visible urine in the urinary bag connected with Foley catheter that was inserted in the neighbourhood clinic he visited prior to current admission. In the clinic, he received 500 ml of 0.9% Saline and another 500 ml was on flow during the process of transfer.

### *13.1.1 What Is the Current Evidence Supporting Fluid Management in Diarrhoeal Illness?*

Diarrhoeal illnesses are common causes of morbidity, need for hospitalization and mortality especially in low- and



S. Ghosh, *Handbook of Intravenous Fluids*,
https://doi.org/10.1007/978-981-19-0500-1_13

middle-income countries and more so in paediatric age group. In fact, according to WHO estimates diarrhoeal diseases are the second leading cause of death in children worldwide (respiratory illnesses leading the list). Between 3 and 6 litres of fluid is secreted from the gastrointestinal tract daily. However, majority of these secreted fluids are being reabsorbed, leaving only 100–200 ml of fluid to be excreted through stool. Profound volume depletion can occur if the reabsorption of fluid is impaired because of pathological processes, like direct bacterial or viral invasion of gastrointestinal tract or toxins, resulting in diarrhoea. Fluid loss can be compensated by increased oral intake (by activation of thirst centre) especially in milder illnesses. However, in more severe illnesses or in patients with refractory vomiting and inability to increase oral intake, develops severe dehydration and evidence of peripheral circulatory failure ("**Hypovolemic Shock**") requiring in-hospital management. Much of the evidence supporting fluid management strategy is derived from paediatric literature. In this chapter, we shall be discussing fluid management strategies in diarrhoeal illness based on physiological rationale and evidence available in paediatric literature.

## 13.2 Diagnosis

- Diagnosis of hypovolemia is obvious from the history itself. However, physical examination and laboratory investigations are useful for understanding degree of dehydration and associated organ dysfunction.
- Physical examination findings that are notable in patients with dehydration ("a term used to describe loss of overall fluid volume in the body including both intra- and extracellular volume to a variable extent") are dry mucus membrane (may be misleading in mouth breathers), decreased skin turgor (misleading in elderly), sunken eyes (especially in children but also in adults in later stage), sunken anterior fontanelles (in infants), low jugular venous pulse, low volume pulse, tachycardia and hypotension.

- Physical findings pointing towards hypovolemic shock are cold extremities with prolonged capillary refill time (CRT), mottled skin, thready pulse, tachycardia, rapid and shallow breathing (due to metabolic acidosis), altered sensorium, hypotension and decreased urine output.
- Laboratory investigations that are most useful during the process of resuscitation are serum electrolytes (especially sodium and potassium), blood glucose and serum lactate (easily available from blood gas machine). Arterial blood gas sampling may be useful to understand degree of metabolic acidosis (or even alkalosis in some cases). Other investigations are directed towards aetiology of diarrhoea (stool examination including culture, blood culture, etc.) or to identify associated organ dysfunction e.g. blood urea nitrogen, serum creatinine to identify renal involvement.
- A simple schema suggested for categorizing degree of dehydration and identifying fluid deficit in children is given in Table 13.1 [1]. This may be useful to some extent in adult patients too.

## 13.3 Management of Dehydration

- Dehydration is the most important adverse consequence of diarrhoeal illnesses and if allowed to remain untreated it may lead to hypovolemic shock, multiple organ failure and eventually death.

### *13.3.1 Which Fluid?*

- Undoubtedly, oneof the greatest medical advances of the twentieth century is the discovery of Oral Rehydration Solution (ORS). ORS solutions are special fluid formulations containing organic substances that are absorbed from the gastrointestinal tract via active co-transport (e.g. glucose or certain amino acids) PLUS sodium chloride, with or without buffering substances.

TABLE 13.1 Classification schema for dehydration severity

| Variable | Mild, 3–5% | Moderate, 6–9% | Severe, >10% |
|---|---|---|---|
| Blood pressure | Normal | Normal | Normal to reduced |
| Pulse quality | Normal | Normal or slightly decreased | Moderately decreased |
| Heart rate | Normal | Increased | Increased |
| Skin turgor | Normal | Decreased | Decreased |
| Fontanelle | Normal | Sunken | Sunken |
| Mucous membrane | Slightly dry | Dry | Dry |
| Eyes | Normal | Sunken orbits | Deeply sunken orbits |
| Extremities | Warm. Normal CRT | Delayed CRT | Cool, mottled |
| Mental status | Normal | Normal to listless | Lethargic to unconscious |
| Urine output | Slightly decreased | <1 ml/kg/h | <<1 ml/kg/h |
| Thirst | Slightly increased | Moderately increased | Very thirsty or too lethargic to indicate |

- Presence of organic substances helps in absorption of sodium and chloride further.
- WHO ORS solution consists of Sodium chloride (2.6 g), Glucose (13.5 g). Potassium Chloride (1.5 g) and Trisodium Citrate Dehydrate (2.9 g) to be dissolved in 1 litre of clean drinking water.
- Overall, electrolyte composition of current WHO ORS solution is given in Table 13.2. There are several other ORS solutions available commercially with more or less similar composition.

Table 13.2 Composition of WHO ORS solution

| | |
|---|---|
| Sodium | 75 mmol/L |
| Chloride | 65 mmol/L |
| Potassium | 20 mmol/L |
| Glucose | 75 mmol/L |
| Citrate | 10 mmol/L |
| Osmolality | 245 mmol/L |

- In a systematic review of 17 clinical trials comparing Oral Rehydration Therapy (ORT) using ORS solution with Intravenous Rehydration Therapy (IRT) in children with acute gastroenteritis associated dehydration [2], there was no difference in overall fluid intake at 6-hour and at 24-hour or weight gain at discharge. Mean duration of diarrhoea was same in two groups. There was no differences in the incidence of hypo- or hypernatraemia
  - ORT was also associated with shorter hospital stays and lower incidence of phlebitis compared to IRT [2].
  - However, ORT was associated with a 4% higher risk of failure to rehydrate. Incidence of paralytic ileus was also higher in ORT group.
- In children with severe dehydration, provision of ORT, at least initially, through nasogastric route achieved similar rate of rehydration compared to IRT [3, 4]. Rate of complications was not different including electrolyte disturbances, fluid overload or abdominal distention. Moreover, duration of diarrhoea was shorter in ORT group.
- Based on the available evidence, in vast majority of patients, dehydration can be treated effectively with ORT using ORS solution. In patients with vomiting, ORT can be tried through nasogastric tube.
- However, intravenous rehydration therapy must be administered in the following situations (choice of intravenous

fluid is discussed in following section on Hypovolaemic Shock):

- Evidence of hypovolemic shock (discussed later in the chapter)
- Failure to rehydrate the patient after initial attempts because of refractory diarrhoea or inability to provide adequate ORT because of profound vomiting
- Evidence of paralytic ileus
- Electrolyte disturbances not getting corrected with ORT alone

- Patients should continue with normal diet, clear liquids, fruit juices during rehydration process as much as possible.
- Those patients who are started on IRT should be re-assessed periodically and should be encouraged to start ORT as soon as possible along with IRT.

### *13.3.2 How Much Fluid?*

- In adult patients, ORS solutions should be administered at lib with periodic monitoring for adequacy and any complications.
- In children, water deficit can be calculated based on the level of dehydration as suggested in Table 13.1.
  - Usually, the calculated deficit is between 50 and 100 ml/Kg body weight and the same deficit should be delivered within 4 h.
  - In cases of vomiting, ORT should be held and should be restarted after 10 min at a slower rate.
- In infants, breastfeeding should be continued throughout the period of rehydration.

### *13.3.3 What to Monitor?*

- Patients should be monitored periodically for the following parameters.

- Amount of ORS solution taken and any other fluid intake.
- Record the number of diarrhoea stools passed or episodes of vomiting.
- Any worsening of dehydration (e.g. further loss of skin turgor, increasing lethargy, decreasing urine output) or increasing stool output.
- Evidence of overhydration like puffy eyelids in children.
- Periodically check electrolytes, e.g. sodium and potassium levels.

## 13.4 Management of Hypovolemic Shock

- In the presence of shock, the primary aim is quick restoration of the tissue perfusion with rapid expansion of intravascular volume and this can be achieved most predictively by intravenous fluid.

### *13.4.1 Which Fluid?*

- There is no head-to-head comparison between different intravenous formulations to be used in hypovolemic shock. However, the following recommendations can be made based on physiological rationale and clinical data from other situations:
  - There is no added advantage of colloid infusions in hypovolemic shock and should be avoided. Though 4% Albumin infusion is found to be safe in SAFE study, it only adds to the cost [5]. In clinical trials conducted in patients with septic shock, hydroxyethyl starch solutions are found to be associated with increased adverse consequences including increased incidence of renal failure, need for renal replacement therapy, need for increased blood products and even increased mortality [6–8].
  - 0.9% Saline is widely available and can be used for initial resuscitation. However, its low strong ion difference may produce metabolic acidosis and high chloride content may be detrimental for renal function.

- Buffered isotonic salt solutions or balanced crystalloids are possibly the best commercially available isotonic crystalloid to be used for resuscitation of hypovolemic shock [9, 10]. Out of all buffered solutions available Lactated Ringer's solution (or Hartman solution) is the most cost-effective ones and is the preferred fluid in WHO guidelines [11].
- Hypotonic solutions (especially only dextrose-containing solutions) should be avoided during resuscitation.

### *13.4.2 How Much Fluid?*

- In the absence of any accurate way of estimating volume deficit, it is prudent to infuse 1–2 litres of isotonic crystalloids as a rapid bolus initially. Decision for subsequent fluid infusion should be guided by the patient's initial response to fluid, evidence of fluid responsiveness and ongoing fluid loss [12].
- Response to fluid can be assessed at the bedside by simple clinical measures like improvement in level of consciousness, return of skin warmth, decreasing CRT, improvement in pulse volume and blood pressure, decrease in heart rate and improvement in urine output.
  - Where available serial measurement of lactate can be useful. Lactate value is expected to show a decreasing trend with improvement in tissue perfusion.
- Ongoing volume loss due to persistent diarrhoea or vomiting must be kept in mind and should be replaced with appropriate fluid ("**Replacement Fluid**").
- Patients should be encouraged to continue their oral intake as much as possible including normal diet, oral rehydration solutions and fruit juices. Carbonated beverages should be avoided.

### *13.4.3 Other Measures*

- Vasopressors should be avoided in hypovolemic shock as they can worsen tissue perfusion.
  - However, in cases of life-threatening hypotension vasopressors should be initiated early.
  - Norepinephrine should be the vasopressor of choice in this situation [13].
  - Vasopressors must be tapered off as early as possible.
- Every effort should be made to establish an etiological diagnosis of diarrhoeal illness especially to look for any treatable condition.
  - Patients with acute watery diarrhoea who are either residing in or who have recently visited cholera endemic areas should be given an appropriate antibiotic once there is no vomiting. Doxycycline is the preferred one in children over 2 years of age and in adults [11]. Other alternative antibiotics for cholera are furazolidone, cotrimoxazole or chloramphenicol. Appropriate use of antibiotics in cholera shortens the duration of diarrhoea.
- In patients with bloody diarrhoea (dysentery), antibiotics must be administered urgently with appropriate coverage for Shigella and Entamoeba [11].

## 13.5 Case Scenario (Continued)

- There is clear evidence of peripheral circulatory failure in Mr. MS due to acute gastroenteritis. Prime aim should be to restore intravascular volume as quickly as possible with intravenous Ringer's lactate—1 to 2 litres initially with subsequent volume decided by frequent monitoring of perfusion parameters.
- Fluids lost due to diarrhoea and vomiting during the period of rehydration should be replaced adequately either by ORS solution administered simultaneously or by Ringer's lactate intravenously.

- He should be encouraged to take normal diet, ORS solutions, clear liquid and fruit juices.
- Considering the clinical scenario and his recent travel to Bengal and coastal Odisha, cholera must be considered as a differential diagnosis and Doxycycline (300 mg) should be administered orally as soon as vomiting settles.

**Take-Home Messages**

- ORS solutions should be administered as soon as possible in patients with dehydration following diarrhoeal illness.
- Intravenous fluid should be infused in patients with hypovolemic shock and those with severe dehydration not responding to initial ORT.

## References

1. Practice parameter: the management of acute gastroenteritis in young children. American Academy of Pediatrics, Provisional Committee on Quality Improvement, Subcommittee on Acute Gastroenteritis. Pediatrics. 1996;97:424–35.
2. Hartling L, Bellemare S, Wiebe N, Russell K, Klassen TP, Craig W. Oral versus intravenous rehydration for treating dehydration due to gastroenteritis in children. Cochrane Database Syst Rev. 2006;2006(3):CD004390.
3. Sharifi J, Ghavami F, Nowrouzi Z, Fouladvand B, Malek M, Rezaeian M, Emami M. Oral versus intravenous rehydration therapy in severe gastroenteritis. Arch Dis Child. 1985;60:856–60.
4. Hidayat S, Srie Enggar KD, Pardede N, Ismail R. Nasogastric drip rehydration therapy in acute diarrhea with severe dehydration. Paediatr Indones. 1988;28:79–84.
5. Finfer S, Bellomo R, Boyce N, French J, Myburgh J, Norton R, SAFE Study Investigators. A comparison of albumin and saline for fluid resuscitation in the intensive care unit. N Engl J Med. 2004;350:2247–56.

6. Brunkhorst FM, Engel C, Bloos F, Meier-Hellmann A, Ragaller M, Weiler N, et al. Intensive insulin therapy and pentastarch resuscitation in severe sepsis. N Engl J Med. 2008;358:125–39.
7. Perner A, Haase N, Guttormsen AB, Tenhunen J, Klemenzson G, Åneman A, et al. Hydroxyethyl starch 130/0.42 versus Ringer's acetate in severe sepsis. N Engl J Med. 2012;367:124–34.
8. Myburgh JA, Finfer S, Bellomo R, Billot L, Cass A, Gattas D, et al. Hydroxyethyl starch or saline for fluid resuscitation in intensive care. N Engl J Med. 2012;367:1901–11.
9. Semler MW, Self WH, Wanderer JP, Ehrenfeld JM, Wang L, Byrne DW, et al. Balanced crystalloids versus saline in critically ill adults. N Engl J Med. 2018;378:829–39.
10. Self WH, Semler MW, Wanderer JP, Wang L, Byrne DW, Collins SP, et al. Balanced crystalloids versus saline in noncritically ill adults. N Engl J Med. 2018;378:819–28.
11. World Health Organization. The treatment of diarrhoea: a manual for physicians and other senior health workers. 4th revision. http://apps.who.int/iris/bitstream/10665/43209/1/9241593180.pdf
12. Latta T. Saline venous injection in cases of malignant cholera, performed while in the vapour-bath. Lancet. 1832;19(480):208–9.
13. De Backer D, Biston P, Devriendt J, Madl C, Chochrad D, Aldecoa C, et al. Comparison of dopamine and norepinephrine in the treatment of shock. N Engl J Med. 2010;362:779–89.

# Chapter 14
# Fluid Resuscitation in Burn

## 14.1 Case Vignette

Mrs. X, a 32-year-old female was rescued by the fire department personnel from a house fire. She is now brought to the emergency department almost an hour after the fire started. On examination in the ED, she is of average built, weighing about 60 kg. She is unconscious with GCS—E1M4V1, heart rate 145/min, blood pressure 126/74 mmHg. There is evidence of partial thickness and deep burn involving trunk (Fig. 14.1), both upper arms, buttocks, neck and face with relative sparing of distal upper and lower limbs and genital. Her peripheries are cold to touch with grossly delayed capillary refill time. She is intubated and put on mechanical ventilator support.

### *14.1.1 How Do You Plan to Start Fluid Resuscitation in Patients with Major Burn Injury?*

Most burns are small and can be managed at home or can be treated on outpatient basis. However, extensive burn injuries are major causes of trauma with high short-term mortality and morbidities, as well as long-term physical, social and economic consequences. Extensive burn injuries produce "**Burn Shock**", characterized by an increase in capillary per-



S. Ghosh, *Handbook of Intravenous Fluids*,
https://doi.org/10.1007/978-981-19-0500-1_14

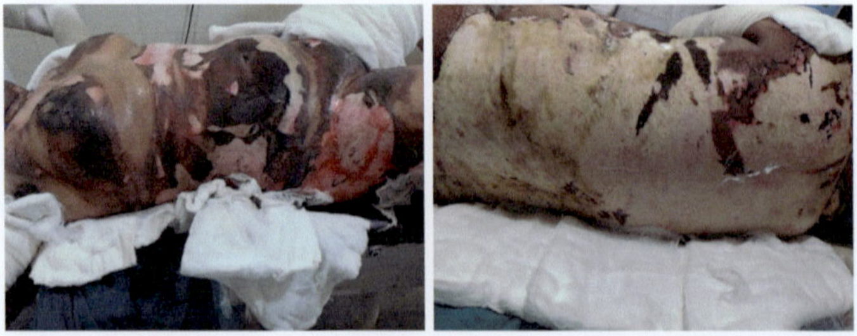

FIGURE 14.1 Clinical photograph (Representative only) showing front and back of a similar patient (taken at a later date) (Photograph Courtesy: Dr. Gaurav Bhatia, MS, MCH, Consultant Plastic Surgeon)

meability, profound depletion of intravascular volume and impaired peripheral perfusion. "Burn shock" requires aggressive and expert fluid resuscitation especially in the first 24 h. Fluid resuscitation should be just adequate as both under and over resuscitation is associated with adverse consequences. In this chapter, we shall discuss the pathophysiology of "burn shock", principles of fluid management in burn including initial fluid planning and monitoring of fluid therapy and complications associated with over resuscitation.

## 14.2 Pathophysiology of Burn Shock

- Extensive thermal injury produces disruption of the transmembrane potential of cells, even those from non-injured areas, resulting in increased intracellular sodium and shift of fluid from intravascular to intracellular compartment.
  - This transmembrane disruption lasts for a few days.
- Tissue injury also activates inflammatory mediators including complement proteins, histamine, prostaglandins, serotonins and kinins. These inflammatory mediators, cause damage to endothelial cells and capillary leak resulting in loss of intravascular fluid, electrolytes and plasma proteins

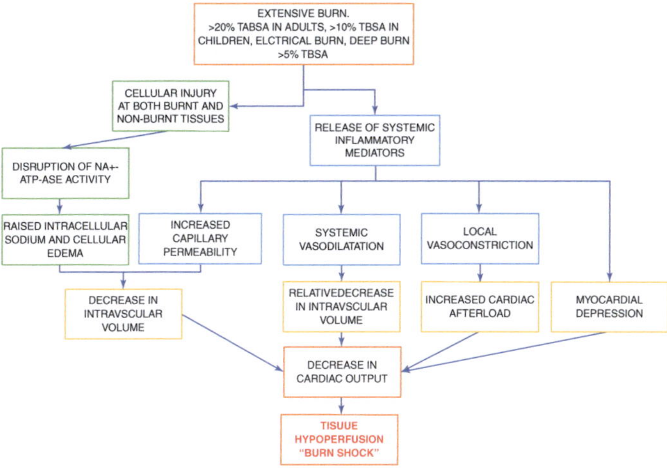


FIGURE 14.2 Pathophysiology of "Burn Shock". *TBSA* total body surface area

to interstitial compartment producing extensive interstitial oedema.

  – Capillary leak reaches its peak 8–12 h after the injury and then gradually improves over 24 to 36 h.

- Inflammatory mediators also lead to both vasodilatation in some vascular beds producing relative hypovolemia and local vasoconstriction producing increased afterload.
- Inflammatory mediators released may also result in myocardial inhibition. Combination of intravascular volume loss (hypovolemia), vasodilatation and myocardial inhibition lead to decrease in cardiac output and tissue hypoperfusion—"**BURN SHOCK**" (Fig. 14.2).

## 14.3 Initial Evaluation

- Like any other emergency, evaluation of burn victims also starts with airway, breathing and circulation.

  - Patients with low GCS ≤8 (because of associated head injury, intoxication, carbon monoxide or cyanide toxicity) or patients with suspected inhalational injury (facial burn, burns sustained in a close-space, singed nasal hair, soot in the oral cavity or throat) need urgent endotracheal intubation.
  - Patients with smoke inhalation or lung injury from inhalation also require ventilatory support.
- During the process of clinical evaluation following aspects should be considered.

### *14.3.1 Estimation of Burn Area*

- In adults, the most popular way to calculate total body surface area (TBSA) of burn is by following "rule of nine".
  - Superficial epidermal burns are not considered for calculation of burn area.
  - According to the "rule of nine", head/neck and each arm (front and back including hand) equal 9% of the body's surface area. Anterior aspect of trunk, back and each leg (front and back including foot) equal 18% of the body's surface area. Groin area equals 1% of the body's surface area.
- Another popular way of estimating the area of burn is by measuring burnt area with patients own palm (excluding fingers)—"rule of palm". The palm of the person is about 1% of the body surface area.
- Burn area > 20% TBSA for adults and > 10% TBSA for children are considered major burn requiring urgent resuscitation.

### *14.3.2 Depth of Burn*

- Depth of burn can be estimated clinically (Table 14.1). Patient with >5% full-thickness burn needs urgent attention [1].

TABLE 14.1 Depth of burn

| Burn type | Appearance | Blisters | Capillary refill | Sensation |
|---|---|---|---|---|
| Epidermal | Red, glistening | None | Brisk | Painful |
| Superficial dermal | Pale pink | Small | Brisk | Painful |
| Deep dermal | Dry, blotchy cherry red | May be present | Absent | Dull or absent |
| Full thickness | Dry, white or black | None | Absent | Absent |

### *14.3.3 Specific Area of Burn*

- Burn patients with involvement of specific areas like hands, face or genitals require specialized care and should be referred to a referral centre as early as feasible.

### *14.3.4 Underlying Conditions*

- Patients with underlying cardiac or respiratory illness need specific attention during resuscitation process and afterwards.

## 14.4 Fluid Resuscitation

- Cornerstone of burn resuscitation is correction of intravascular volume without causing undue harm from overloading the patient.
- Multiple formulas have been described for burn resuscitation. They take into consideration both weight of the patient and percentage of total body surface area burnt (as calculated by "rule of nine") and give an estimation for initial rate of fluid resuscitation.
- Two of the popular formulas are "Parkland Formula" and "modified Brooke Formula".

### 14.4.1 Parkland Formula

- It recommends 4 ml/kg body weight/%TBSA to be infused in the first 24 h in the form of Ringer's Lactate with half the calculated volume to be administered in the first 8 h post-burn and remaining half over the next 16-h.
  - Example. For a 70 kg patient with 60% burn initial calculated resuscitation fluid volume for first 24-h would be 4 mL × 70 × 60 = 16,800 ml. Out of this calculated volume, 8400 ml would be infused in the first 8 h. Hence, the initial rate of resuscitation will be 1 litre/h of Ringer's Lactate.
- For paediatric patients, the Parkland Formula can be used with an addition of normal maintenance fluids added to the volume calculated by the formula.

### 14.4.2 Modified Brooke Formula

- This formula proposes administration of Ringer's Lactate at a rate of 2 ml/kg body weight/%TBSA to be infused in the first 24 h post-burn.
- In a study of 52 patients with major burn, resuscitated with either Parkland or modified Brooke formula, Chung and colleagues did not find any major outcome differences between the two groups [2].
- American Burn Association guideline recommends 2–4 ml/Kg/%TBSA over 24-h as the starting rate of resuscitation [3].

## 14.5 Monitoring

- During the process of resuscitation, burn victims should be monitored periodically to ensure adequacy of resuscitation as well as to avoid over-resuscitation.
- Hourly urine output is the most widely accepted monitoring tool during burn resuscitation. Guideline suggests

urine output goal of 0.5–1 ml/kg/h or approximately 30–50 ml/h for adults and 1–2 ml/kg/h for children, with an increase in rate of fluid infusion if the output falls below 30 ml/h for few hours [3]. Conversely, if the output goes beyond 50 ml/h for a few hours, infusion rate should be decreased to avoid over-resuscitation.

- Other basic monitoring tools to be utilized at the bedside are sensorium, blood pressure, heart rate, haemoglobin/haematocrit, lactate and base excess.
- Central venous pressure (CVP), pulmonary capillary wedge pressure (PCWP) or parameters to monitor fluid responsiveness are suggested by researchers to optimize preload and restore cardiac output.
  - In a randomized control study, 50 patients with >20% TBSA burn were resuscitated with either Parkland formula or thermodilution (TDD) catheter-guided strategy. Despite receiving a significantly higher resuscitation volume (>11 litre in first 24 h), cardiac output goal could not be achieved in TDD group [4].
  - Guideline does not recommend routine monitoring of preload parameters or cardiac output during initial period of resuscitation with the exception of elderly patients or patients with cardiopulmonary compromise or in patients with inadequate response to initial resuscitation [3].
- A suggested approach to monitoring resuscitation of burn victims during their intensive care unit stay is given in Table 14.2.

## 14.6 Fluid Creep

- Burn patients too often receive more resuscitation volume than predicted by formulas. Dr. Basil Pruitt coined the term "**Fluid Creep**" to describe this phenomenon [5].
- Fluid creep can potentially lead to an increase in interstitial oedema, increased pressure in close compartments (including raised intra-abdominal pressure, intra-ocular pressure, pressure in limb compartments), compromise

Table 14.2 Monitoring strategies during resuscitation of patients with major burn

| Early < 24 h | Late > 24 h | Late refractory |
|---|---|---|
| • Fluid is lifesaving.<br>• Liberal fluid administration. | • Fluid is a biomarker.<br>• Maintain euvolemia. | • Fluid is toxic.<br>• Avoid excess.<br>• Goal-directed fluid removal. |
| • Basic monitoring.<br>• May consider using:<br>- Invasive blood pressure.<br>- Ultrasonography.<br>- Cardiac output monitoring for high-risk patients. | • Basic monitoring.<br>• May consider using:<br>- Fluid responsiveness parameters.<br>- Ultrasonography.<br>- Cardiac output monitoring. | • Basic monitoring.<br>• May consider using:<br>- Extravascular lung water.<br>- Lung ultrasonography. |

blood flow to tissue/organs and produce tissue/organ dysfunction (including abdominal compartment syndrome, acute kidney injury, damage to optic nerve or muscles of extremities) [6]. Some of the important points pertaining to the phenomenon of "Fluid Creep" are described below.

I. Increased requirement of resuscitation volume is associated with an increased risk of complications.
   - But the relationship between the rate of complications and infusion volume is not linear, especially for abdominal compartment syndrome and raised intraocular pressure, unless the total volume exceeds "**Ivy Index**" of >250 ml/kg/%Total Body Surface Area (TBSA) burn [7–9].
   - This may simply mean that, at least for some patients, increased requirement of resuscitation volume is a normal phenomenon.

II. Fluid requirements for burn increases disproportionately with larger area of burn injury [10].

III. Subgroup of patients with burn injury requires larger volume of resuscitation fluid.

- In their original report, Baxter and colleagues noted that patients with delayed presentation, deeper burn and inhalation injury certainly require more fluids than predicted [11].

IV. Opioid infusions to relieve pain produces vasodilatation and hypotension. This may lead to resuscitation with more fluid. Sullivan and colleagues described this phenomenon as "**Opioid Creep**" [12].

V. Burn resuscitation that begins with higher planned resuscitation volume ends up receiving more fluid—"fluid begets more fluid".

- This phenomenon was clearly demonstrated by Chung and colleagues examining US military burn causalities. They observed that these patients despite having similar baseline characteristics received significantly more fluid when they are started on the Parkland formula (4 ml/kg/%TBSA burn) compared to modified Brooke's formula (2 ml/kg/%TBSA burn) [2].
- This is possibly related to initial crystalloid volumes getting accumulated in the interstitial compartment in the initial period of resuscitation and changing its collagen-hyaluronic acid matrix [6].

VI. Initial resuscitation rate needs to be titrated against hourly urine output of the patient with an increase in rate of infusion with a fall in urine output and vice versa. However, studies have shown that clinicians are less likely to reduce infusion volume in the presence of increased urine output, potentially contributing to "fluid creep" [10].

VII. Current trend towards "goal-directed resuscitation" in critical care targeting cardiac output or clearing of lactate may also be contributing to increased and unnecessary resuscitation volume [6].

## 14.7 Managing Fluid Creep

- Keeping in mind diverse aetiologies of "Fluid Creep", all resuscitation protocol must be flexible, so that it can deal with all the issues described in the previous section. Following modalities can be helpful in either preventing or reversing the progression of the problem.

  I. **Reduced initial rate of infusion:** As seen by Chung and colleagues, lower initial infusion rate can potentially reduce overall "Fluid Creep" [2].

     – Another potential way is to avoid usual "knee jerk response" to hypotension—giving fluid boluses to correct it [6]. Hypotension is more likely because of the injury itself and usually nothing to do with status of resuscitation.

  II. **Adhering to the Target Urine Output:** Reduce the infusion rate, if the urine output exceeds the target.

  III. **Permissive Hypoperfusion:** In a single-centre study of paediatric patients with 15% TBSA scald burn, resuscitation was initiated with rate of 2 mL/kg/%TBSA plus 80% maintenance fluid requirement calculated [13]. Urine output goal was set at 0.5 ml/kg/h (compared to the aim of 1 ml/kg/h as suggested by guideline) as long as these children remained clinically well perfused and they were not acidotic.

     – Compared to the control group (i.e. historical patient cohort from the same centre and patients from surrounding centres treated using standard guidelines), patients in permissive hypoperfusion group had a lower rate of ICU admission, lower length of stay without any increase in renal dysfunction or depth of burn [13].
     – However, results of this study need to be validated in other centres with larger area of burn and in adult population, before its widespread application.

IV. **Judicious use of colloids:** In the initial 8–12 h of resuscitation when the capillary permeability is high, infusion of colloid is unlikely to be helpful. But after 12–18 h infusion of colloid may be helpful both for prevention of fluid creep and also as a rescue therapy for the same [6].

- Albumin is the most widely used colloid for this purpose. In a recent systematic review, albumin infusion had shown to reduce mortality and decrease occurrence of compartment syndrome [14].
- One suggested approach is to calculate the projected 24-h resuscitation volume, after initial 12 to 18 h of fluid infusion and to start 5% Albumin infusion, if the projected volume exceeds 6 ml/kg/%TBSA [15].
- Another option is to utilise fresh frozen plasma (FFP). In a randomized control trial, resuscitation with FFP was shown to be associated with reduced infusion volume and reduced increase in intra-abdominal pressure compared to crystalloid resuscitation [16]. But these beneficial effects of FFP need to be weighed against the potential adverse effects like transmission of blood-borne pathogens, cost and transfusion-associated acute lung injury (TRALI).
- Hydroxyethyl starch and other synthetic colloids should be avoided in of their known association with increased mortality, acute kidney injury and coagulopathy in septic shock resuscitation.

V. **Hypertonic Saline:** Hypertonic saline solution has been suggested as a potential mean to reduce resuscitation volume and fluid creep. However, same strategy has not been demonstrated in any randomized study till date [17].

  - Moreover, potential benefit of hypertonic saline should be balanced against the potential for producing hypernatremia and acute kidney injury [6].

VI. **High-dose Ascorbic Acid:** Ascorbic acid has been shown to reduce fluid infusion volume in multiple small studies, possibly tightening the endothelial cell barrier through its effect on endothelial cells.

  - Recent Japanese registry data has shown high-dose ascorbic acid (minimum 10 g in first 2 days after burn) to be associated with reduced mortality in major burn injury [18].

VII. **Plasmapheresis:** In selected cases, plasmapheresis may be used to treat fluid creep and raised abdominal pressure [6].

## 14.8 Case Scenario (Continued)

- The scenario describes a case of major burn with %TBSA of approximately 55% (head and neck—9%, chest and abdomen—18%, back—18%, proximal upper limbs (both)—9%).
- Possible causes of unconsciousness in Mrs. X could be because of intoxication or associated head injury or because of toxic gas inhalation (carbon monoxide or cyanide toxicity) or inhalation injury causing type 2 Respiratory failure. She required urgent endotracheal intubation both in view of low GCS and possible inhalation injury (facial burn).
- Her initial investigations should include complete blood count especially haemoglobin/haematocrit, arterial blood gas including co-oximetry (to look for oxygenation status, pH, base excess, partial pressure of $CO_2$, lactate and level of carboxyhaemoglobin), kidney function tests including electrolytes, blood glucose, creatine kinase to look for evidence of potential rhabdomyolysis and urine analysis including urine pH. Screening should be done to rule out other injuries including CT head.

- Fluid resuscitation should be started immediately. Calculated fluid volume for the first 24 h using Parkland Formula is $4 \times 60 \times 55 = 13{,}200$ ml. With 6600 ml Ringer's Lactate to be infused over the next 7 h (patient had arrived in the ED with a delay of 1 h) initial rate of resuscitation should be approximately 950 ml/h. Fluid infusion rate should be modified if necessary in subsequent hours based on hourly urine output.

**Take-Home Messages**

- Infusion with crystalloid (Ringer's Lactate) is the cornerstone of burn resuscitation. Initial rate of infusion should be calculated based on well-accepted formula like Parkland or modified Brooke.
- Initial infusion rate should be adjusted based on urine output target.
- Invasive hemodynamic monitoring is advisable in high-risk patients and in patients who have failed to respond to initial resuscitation.
- Fluid creep is common and should be looked for during the resuscitation process. Albumin infusion starting at 12–18 h for patients with an expected 14-h resuscitation volume exceeding 6 ml/kg/%TBSA is a potential way to reduce fluid creep.

## References

1. Enoch S, Roshan A, Shah M. Emergency and early management of burns and scalds. BMJ. 2009;338:b1037.
2. Chung KK, Wolf SE, Cancio LC, Alvarado R, Jones JA, McCorcle J, et al. Resuscitation of severely burned military casualties: fluid begets more fluid. J Trauma. 2009;67:231–7.
3. Pham TN, Cancio LC, Gibran NS, American Burn Association. American burn association practice guidelines burn shock resuscitation. J Burn Care Res. 2008;29:257–66.

4. Holm C, Mayr M, Tegeler J, Hörbrand F, Henckel von Donnersmarck G, Mühlbauer W, Pfeiffer UJ. A clinical randomized study on the effects of invasive monitoring on burn shock resuscitation. Burns. 2004;30:798–807.
5. Pruitt BA Jr. Protection from excessive resuscitation: "pushing the pendulum back". J Trauma. 2000 Sep;49(3):567–8.
6. Saffle JR. Fluid creep and over-resuscitation. Crit Care Clin. 2016;32:587–98.
7. Klein MB, Hayden D, Elson C, Nathens AB, Gamelli RL, Gibran NS, et al. The association between fluid administration and outcome following major burn: a multicentre study. Ann Surg. 2007;245:622–8.
8. Ivy ME, Atweh NA, Palmer J, Possenti PP, Pineau M, D'Aiuto M. Intra-abdominal hypertension and abdominal compartment syndrome in burn patients. J Trauma. 2000;49:387–91.
9. Markell KW, Renz EM, White CE, Albrecht ME, Blackbourne LH, Park MS, et al. Abdominal complications after severe burns. J Am Coll Surg. 2009;208:940–7.
10. Cancio LC, Chávez S, Alvarado-Ortega M, Barillo DJ, Walker SC, McManus AT, Goodwin CW. Predicting increased fluid requirements during the resuscitation of thermally injured patients. J Trauma. 2004;56:404–13.
11. Baxter CR. Problems and complications of burn shock resuscitation. Surg Clin North Am. 1978;58:1313–22.
12. Sullivan SR, Friedrich JB, Engrav LH, Round KA, Heimbach DM, Heckbert SR, et al. "Opioid creep" is real and may be the cause of "fluid creep". Burns. 2004;30:583–90.
13. Walker TL, Rodriguez DU, Coy K, Hollén LI, Greenwood R, Young AE. Impact of reduced resuscitation fluid on outcomes of children with 10-20% body surface area scalds. Burns. 2014;40:1581–6.
14. Navickis RJ, Greenhalgh DG, Wilkes MM. Albumin in burn shock resuscitation: a meta-analysis of controlled clinical studies. J Burn Care Res. 2016;37:e268–78.
15. Chung KK, Blackbourne LH, Wolf SE, White CE, Renz EM, Cancio LC, Holcomb JB, Barillo DJ. Evolution of burn resuscitation in operation Iraqi freedom. J Burn Care Res. 2006;27:606–11.
16. O'Mara MS, Slater H, Goldfarb IW, Caushaj PF. A prospective, randomized evaluation of intra-abdominal pressures with crystalloid and colloid resuscitation in burn patients. J Trauma. 2005;58:1011–8.

17. Huang PP, Stucky FS, Dimick AR, Treat RC, Bessey PQ, Rue LW. Hypertonic sodium resuscitation is associated with renal failure and death. Ann Surg. 1995;221:543–54.
18. Nakajima M, Kojiro M, Aso S, Matsui H, Fushimi K, Kaita Y, et al. Effect of high-dose vitamin C therapy on severe burn patients: a nationwide cohort study. Crit Care. 2019;23:407.

# Chapter 15
# Fluid Management in Perioperative Period

## 15.1 Case Scenario

Mrs. AS, a 46-year-old female patient was recently diagnosed to have a lump in her right breast. Tissue biopsy confirmed carcinoma breast and staging investigations showed involvement of unilateral axillary lymph nodes in the right side. She is now admitted to the surgical wards with a planned right-sided radical mastectomy under general anaesthesia on the following day. She denies any other co-morbid illness. She is of medium build, weighing 60 kg. There is no clinical evidence of hypovolemia.

### *15.1.1 What Should Be the Optimal Fluid Management Strategy for Surgical Patients in the Peri-operative Period?*

Optimal management of perioperative fluid plays an important role in the postoperative recovery of surgical patients. Major surgeries produce significant changes in the fluid status of the patient because of various factors including evaporative loss from open wound, shifting of fluid from intravascular to interstitial compartments, underlying disease



S. Ghosh, *Handbook of Intravenous Fluids*,
https://doi.org/10.1007/978-981-19-0500-1_15

process itself, systemic inflammatory response syndrome and intra-/postoperative blood loss. The extent of these changes varies, based on several factors including types of surgery (abdominal or extra-abdominal or vascular), surgical techniques (open or laparoscopic or robotic), skill and tissue handling by surgeon, emergency nature of the surgery, type of anaesthesia and finally patient-related factors (physiological status, co-morbidities). Goal is to maintain tissue perfusion and to avoid organ damage (by avoiding both hypovolemia and hypotension) without producing iatrogenic tissue oedema that can impair tissue healing, cause wound dehiscence, promote infection, pulmonary oedema and other myriad complications.

Three major strategies are described for perioperative fluid management each having its own advantages and limitations: "**Standard Approach**", "**Restricted Approach**" (or so-called "**Zero Balance Approach**") and "**Goal-Directed Approach**" [1]. Another aspect to consider in perioperative fluid management is the inter-related but apparently separate fluid management strategies in preoperative, intraoperative and postoperative periods. In this chapter, we shall discuss three different strategies of perioperative fluid management including their current evidence and shall suggest an approach for pre-, intra- and postoperative periods. We shall also have a brief discussion on the types of fluid to be prescribed keeping in mind both "maintenance fluid" and "resuscitation/replacement fluid".

## 15.2 Standard Approach

- Standard approach, as suggested in some textbooks, proposes a strategy to replace fluid losses in the perioperative periods including the loss to so-called "**Third Space**" [2].
  - Third space is defined as the fluid volume that shifted from the intravascular to interstitial compartment during perioperative period.

- Number of empirical formulae have been suggested to calculate this third space loss of fluid, based on duration and type of surgery and amount of tissue handling.

- Standard strategy results in postoperative weight gain to the tune of 3–6 kg.
- However, hypovolemia from this presumed third spacing does not occur in all patients on a regular basis. Hence, fluid loading to correct third space loss based on empirical formulae is not justifiable especially in otherwise healthy patients and in patients undergoing low-intensity surgery. This can only lead to intravascular hypervolemia, release of atrial natriuretic peptides resulting in degradation of glycocalyx and increase in vascular permeability, tissue oedema and organ dysfunction.

## 15.3 Restricted Approach

- In this approach, all measurable fluid losses plus fluid lost because of sweating, evaporation and respiration (or "Insensible Loss") are replaced appropriately with a goal to maintain zero fluid balance. In this approach, no attempt is made to replace fluid lost to "third space".
  - Restricted approach aims at reduction of positive fluid balance, avoiding harmful effects of interstitial oedema on tissue healing, cardiovascular and pulmonary function.
- In a multicentre Danish study, Brandstrup and colleagues randomized 172 patients undergoing colorectal surgery to one of the two perioperative fluid management strategies—restricted strategy aiming to maintain preoperative weight of the patient or standard approach [3].
  - In the restricted approach, preloading before epidural analgesia and fluid replacement for supposed third-space loss were avoided completely. In the postopera-

tive period, weight gain in excess of 1 kg was treated with diuretics.

  - Restricted group received a significantly lower volume of intravenous fluid on the day of surgery (2740 ml vs. 5388 ml) [3]. Intravenous fluid volume was also lesser on first postoperative day in the restricted group.
  - Throughout the first six postoperative days, patients in the restricted group had significantly lower body weight compared to the standard group.
  - Both cardiopulmonary and tissue-healing complications were significantly reduced in the restricted fluid group without any increase in harmful adverse effects [3]. Compared to four deaths in the standard group, no death was observed in the restricted group.

- In a systematic review of nine studies comparing "restricted" versus "standard or liberal" approaches to perioperative fluid management, authors found a significantly lower rate of complications and shorter hospital length of stay in patients who received fluid in a balanced way, closer to achieving zero fluid balance [4].
- However, too stringent restriction of fluid may not be desirable in all patients. In a multicentre RELIEF study, 3000 patients undergoing major abdominal surgery were randomized to restricted or liberal strategy [5].

  - At 24 h, the restricted group received 3.7 litres of fluid compared to 6.1 litres in liberal group; resulting in an increase in body weight by 0.3 kg and 1.6 kg, respectively, in two groups at 24 h. Intraoperative fluid volume administered in restricted and liberal groups were 1.7 litres and 3 litres, respectively.
  - There was no difference in primary outcome, i.e. disability-free survival at one year. However, the incidence of acute kidney injury was significantly higher in restricted group.
  - There were significant drawbacks to the postoperative fluid management strategy in these trials, as pointed out in the accompanying editorial [6]. No specific strategy

was in place in cases of oliguria, hypovolemia was treated only in cases of blood loss and episodes of hypotension were treated with vasopressor. This insufficient access to adequate fluid possibly led to increased incidences of acute kidney injury [5].

## 15.4 Goal-Directed Approach

- The goal-directed approach is based on the concept of making a right balance between increased oxygen demand during surgery and maintaining tissue perfusion, by using basic and advanced hemodynamic parameters.
  - Aim of goal-directed approach is to maintain targeted hemodynamic endpoints (either flow or pressure or both) rather than a predetermined perioperative fluid balance and thus individualizing administration of perioperative intravenous fluid.
- In the multicentre OPTIMISE study from the United Kingdom, 734 patients undergoing major gastrointestinal surgery were randomized to cardiac output-guided hemodynamic therapy algorithm utilizing both intravenous fluid and inotropes or to usual care [7].
  - There was a strong trend towards a lower incidence of moderate to major complications and mortality at 30 days (Primary Outcome) favouring intervention group (36.6% vs. 43.4%). However, the difference was not statistically significant.
  - A meta-analysis that accompanied the study (total of 38 trials including data from OPTIMISE), however, showed a significantly lower risk of complications (31.5% vs. 41.6%) and mortality (8.3% vs. 10.3%) in goal-directed fluid therapy group [7].
- In the Spanish multicentre FEDORA study, 450 patients undergoing major abdominal, urological, gynaecological or orthopaedic surgery under general anaesthesia were

randomized to goal-directed fluid management group in whom intraoperative administration of fluids, inotropes and vasopressors were guided by stroke volume, cardiac index (measured by oesophageal Doppler) and mean arterial pressure or to usual care group in whom moderate restriction of fluid administration was followed intraoperatively [8].

- According to the algorithm, fluid status was first optimized to maximize stroke volume, followed by the addition of vasopressor or inotrope (as needed) to maintain mean arterial pressure > 65 mm Hg and cardiac index greater than 2.5 litre/min/$m^2$.
- Major surgery was defined as those with an expected duration of at least 2 h with estimated blood loss >15% of blood volume or transfusion requirement of at least two packed red blood cells.
- Moderate to severe postoperative complications were significantly lower in the goal-directed group (8.6% vs. 16.6%).
- Incidences of acute kidney injury, pulmonary oedema, acute respiratory distress syndrome and wound infections were also lower in the intervention group [8].

- In the multicentre, French IMPRESS study, an individualized fluid management strategy aiming to achieve intraoperative and up to 4 h postoperative systolic blood pressure (SBP) within 10% of the patient's resting value was found to reduce incidences of systemic inflammatory response syndrome or organ dysfunction at 7 days, compared to standard strategy of only treating SBP less than 80 mmHg [9].

## 15.5 Making a Balance

- In perioperative fluid management, both "Restricted Approach" and "Goal-Directed Approach" have clearly shown superiority compared to "Standard Approach" [4, 10].

- In a multicentre Danish study, goal-directed strategy aiming for a near-maximal stroke volume guided by oesophageal Doppler was compared with restrictive approach aiming for a zero balance or a normal body weight, in 150 patients undergoing colorectal surgery [1].
- At 30 days, no significant differences were observed between the two groups in major, minor, cardiopulmonary or tissue healing complications.

- However, best approach possibly will be to make an individualized strategy.
- Considerations should be given to the patient's baseline cardiopulmonary risk and the risk of surgery itself (expected duration, expected blood loss or transfusion requirement, tissue handling like laparoscopic or open).
- Miller and colleagues suggested a balanced approach to perioperative fluid management and is summarized in Fig. 15.1 [11].

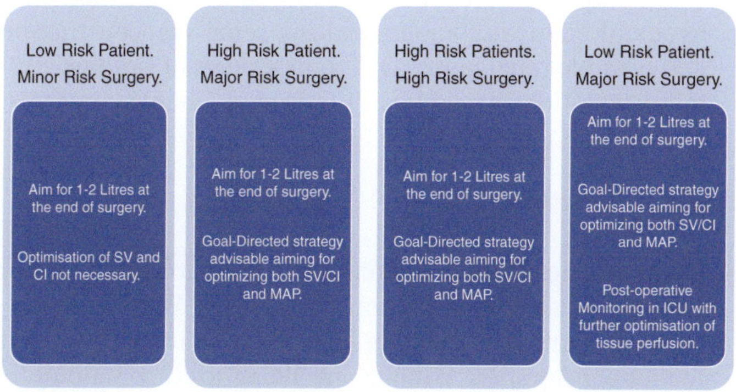


FIGURE 15.1 Making a balance between restricted and goal-directed approach

## 15.6 Which Fluid?

- Intravenous fluids are being used in perioperative setting for either maintenance purposes or as a volume expander for resuscitation or replacement purposes.

### *15.6.1 Maintenance Fluid*

- For most patients moderately, hypotonic dextrose-containing solutions with an adequate concentration of electrolytes (especially sodium, potassium and chloride) should be used for maintenance purposes. In both pre- and postoperative setting. The rationale for this recommendation is discussed in Chap. 7.
- Isotonic crystalloids are possibly the maintenance solution of choice during surgery [11]. Balanced solutions are preferred over 0.9% Saline, as their electrolyte composition more closely resembles concentration in plasma. Moreover, 0.9% Saline is now clearly shown to be associated with hyperchloremic metabolic acidosis, renal vasoconstriction and possible renal injury. Different aspects of isotonic crystalloid solutions have been discussed in Chap. 5.

### *15.6.2 Resuscitation or Volume Therapy*

- Controversies still prevail regarding the choice of fluid for volume therapy in perioperative setting. With a physiologic rationale of remaining in intravascular compartment for longer duration, colloids are being used commonly in this setting. Indeed, in most goal-directed therapy studies and many of the restricted strategy studies, colloids especially hydroxyethyl starch (HES) boluses were used for this purpose [1, 8–10].
- In a meta-analysis, comprising 13 small studies, comparing hydroxyethyl starch and crystalloid solutions in patients undergoing non-cardiac surgery, authors could

demonstrate lower IV fluid volume infusion with HES solutions [12].

 - However, there was a trend towards (statistically non-significant) increased 90-day mortality in HES group (Risk Ratio 2.97; 95% Confidence Interval 0.96 to 9.19).
 - Interestingly, unlike studies in general ICU patients or in patients with sepsis, the analysis failed to show any increase in the incidence of Acute Kidney Injury or need for Renal Replacement Therapy in the HES group [12].

- In a more recent bi-centre study, 160 patients undergoing major elective abdominal surgery receiving goal-directed fluid strategy were randomized to receive either balanced crystalloid (Plasmalyte) or HES in balanced crystalloid (Volulyte) for volume therapy, using a closed-loop system (in 100 ml boluses guided by stroke volume and stroke volume variation) [13].
  - All patients received maintenance balanced crystalloid solution (Plasmalyte). Total intraoperative fluid volume and net fluid balance were significantly lower in HES group.
  - HES group also had lower Postoperative morbidity survey score on day 2 after surgery (Primary Outcome) and lower incidence of postoperative complications [13].
- There are very little data available regarding the use of other synthetic colloids and albumin in perioperative setting. Use of albumin is as such limited, because of cost-concern.
- Overall, colloids (especially HES) versus crystalloid debate continues in perioperative volume therapy. Unlike in general ICU scenarios, HES has not shown a clear increase in morbidity and mortality in this setting and still continued to be used.
  - However, while using HES in this setting one should keep in mind its potential for producing renal injury

and coagulopathy especially in large volume (observed in ICU setting), limited evidence supporting its benefit in true patient-centred outcome and additional cost involved.

- In cases of major bleeding, volume must be replaced by appropriate blood and blood products.

## 15.7 Perioperative Fluid: To Summarize

- A brief overview of suggested strategies is given in Table 15.1. Management of fluid in individual organ-specific surgeries is beyond the scope of this chapter.

## 15.8 Case Scenario (Continued)

- Mrs. AS is planned for a major surgery that is expected to last more than 2 h with not much-anticipated blood loss, under general anaesthesia.
- She should be encouraged to take clear liquid until 2 h before induction of anaesthesia.
- During surgery, she may be maintained on 600–700 ml/h of balanced isotonic crystalloid (e.g. RL or Plasmalyte) infusion. In between, boluses of balanced crystalloid may be administered for hemodynamic optimization and maintenance of systolic blood pressure.
- Postoperatively she should be started on oral feeding as soon as effects of general anaesthesia wane off. Till that time, she may be maintained on moderately hypotonic dextrose-containing solution (e.g. 0.45% Saline plus 5% Dextrose) at a rate of about 90 ml/h.

TABLE 15.1 Summary of perioperative fluid management

| | |
|---|---|
| Preoperative | • Minimize preoperative fasting time.<br>• Encourage clear liquid until 2 h before surgery.<br>• If the patient is not in a position to take orally and enteral route is not available, intravenous maintenance fluid should be prescribed. Moderately hypotonic dextrose-containing fluid is preferred unless there is a risk of raised intracranial pressure. |
| Intraoperative | • All patients should have a hemodynamic and fluid management plan in place. Both hypovolemia and hypotension must be avoided.<br>• In major surgeries (procedure lasting for >2 h or expected to have >15% loss of blood volume or those requiring extensive tissue handling), goal should be to achieve 1–2 litres of positive fluid balance at the end of surgeries.<br>• For other surgeries or in laparoscopic surgeries may be a lower fluid balance is acceptable.<br>• Balanced crystalloids are preferred as maintenance fluid intraoperatively. Initially, maintenance fluid can be started at a rate of 10–12 ml/kg/h, to be titrated based on patient's hemodynamic status and urine output.<br>• Intraoperative volume resuscitation can be done using either balanced crystalloid solutions or hydroxyethyl starch solutions. However, volume of HES used should not exceed manufacturer's recommendation.<br>• Use advanced hemodynamic monitoring for both high-risk patients and patients undergoing major surgery. Goal-directed strategy looking for optimizing both volume status and blood pressure is certainly preferred in such patients.<br>• Use smaller boluses of 100 to 250 ml for volume therapy and to avoid fluid overload.<br>• Optimize volume first before adding vasopressors to maintain systolic blood pressure within 10% of baseline values.<br>• Use blood products early to correct blood loss. |

(continued)

Table 15.1 (continued)

| | |
|---|---|
| Postoperative | • Target early transition from intravenous fluid to oral/enteral feeding [14].<br>• Remove intravenous lines as early as possible.<br>• In case oral/enteral route is not available use hypotonic dextrose containing maintenance fluid, keeping in mind adequate electrolyte replacement.<br>• Maintenance infusion can be provided at a rate of 1.5 ml/kg/h with close monitoring of urine output [11] adequate pain relief must be ensured (pain is a strong stimulus for arginine vasopressin or antidiuretic hormone release from posterior pituitary). |

(*SV* Stroke Volume, *CI* Cardiac Index, *MAP* Mean Arterial Pressure, *ICU* Intensive Care Unit)

**Take-Home Messages**

- A fluid management plan must be in place for every patient undergoing surgery based on type of surgery, type of anaesthesia and patient's baseline physiological status.
- An individualized strategy aiming for a goal-directed optimization of volume status and blood pressure is perhaps preferable. However, an otherwise healthy patient undergoing minor surgeries may not need sophisticated monitoring.
- Practice of fluid replacement strategy targeting so-called third space loss should be abandoned.
- Unless contraindicated patients should be allowed to take clear liquid orally till 2 h before surgery.
- In patients, goal should be to have a positive fluid balance of 1–2 Litres at the end of surgeries.
- Postoperatively oral fluid/feed should be started as early as possible. Both postoperative hypovolemia and hypotension must be avoided.

## References

1. Brandstrup B, Svendsen PE, Rasmussen M, Belhage B, Rodt SA, Hansen B, et al. Which goal for fluid therapy during colorectal surgery is followed by the best outcome: near-maximal stroke volume or zero fluid balance? Br J Anaesth. 2012;109:191–9.
2. McKinlay S, Gan TJ. Intravenous fluid therapy in daily practice: intraabdominal operations. In: Hahn RG, Prough DS, Svensen CH, editors. Perioperative fluid therapy. New York: Informa Healthcare USA, Inc.; 2007. p. 357–64.
3. Brandstrup B, Tønnesen H, Beier-Holgersen R, Hjortsø E, Ørding H, Lindorff-Larsen K, et al. Effects of intravenous fluid restriction on postoperative complications: comparison of two perioperative fluid regimens: a randomized assessor-blinded multicenter trial. Ann Surg. 2003;238:641–8.
4. Varadhan KK, Lobo DN. A meta-analysis of randomised controlled trials of intravenous fluid therapy in major elective open abdominal surgery: getting the balance right. Proc Nutr Soc. 2010;69:488–98.
5. Myles PS, Bellomo R, Corcoran T, Forbes A, Peyton P, Story D, et al. Restrictive versus liberal fluid therapy for major abdominal surgery. N Engl J Med. 2018;378:2263–74.
6. Brandstrup B. Finding the right balance. N Engl J Med. 2018;378:2335–6.
7. Pearse RM, Harrison DA, MacDonald N, Gillies MA, Blunt M, Ackland G, et al. Effect of a perioperative, cardiac output-guided hemodynamic therapy algorithm on outcomes following major gastrointestinal surgery: a randomized clinical trial and systematic review. JAMA. 2014;311:2181–90.
8. Calvo-Vecino JM, Ripollés-Melchor J, Mythen MG, Casans-Francés R, Balik A, Artacho JP, et al. Effect of goal-directed haemodynamic therapy on postoperative complications in low-moderate risk surgical patients: a multicentre randomised controlled trial (FEDORA trial). Br J Anaesth. 2018;120:734–44.
9. Futier E, Lefrant JY, Guinot PG, Godet T, Lorne E, Cuvillon P, et al. Effect of individualized vs standard blood pressure management strategies on postoperative organ dysfunction among high-risk patients undergoing major surgery: a randomized clinical trial. JAMA. 2017;318:1346–57.

10. Messina A, Robba C, Calabrò L, Zambelli D, Lanuzzi F, Molinari E, et al. Association between perioperative fluid administration and postoperative outcomes: a 20-year systematic review and a meta-analysis of randomized goal-directed trials in major visceral/noncardiac surgery. Crit Care. 2021;25:43.
11. Miller TE, Myles PS. Perioperative fluid therapy for major surgery. Anesthesiology. 2019;130:825–32.
12. Raiman M, Mitchell CG, Biccard BM, Rodseth RN. Comparison of hydroxyethyl starch colloids with crystalloids for surgical patients: a systematic review and meta-analysis. Eur J Anaesthesiol. 2016;33:42–8.
13. Joosten A, Delaporte A, Ickx B, Touihri K, Stany I, Barvais L, et al. Crystalloid versus colloid for intraoperative goal-directed fluid therapy using a closed-loop system: a randomized, double-blinded, controlled trial in major abdominal surgery. Anesthesiology. 2018;128:55–66.
14. Feldheiser A, Aziz O, Baldini G, Cox BP, Fearon KC, Feldman LS, et al. Enhanced recovery after surgery (ERAS) for gastrointestinal surgery, part 2: consensus statement for anaesthesia practice. Acta Anaesthesiol Scand. 2016;60:289–334.

# Chapter 16
# Fluid Management in Diabetic Ketoacidosis

## 16.1 Case Scenario

Mrs. AG, a 24-year-lady with a past history of Type 1 Diabetes Mellitus on insulin therapy presented to the emergency department with history of progressive shortness of breath for past 3 days and altered sensorium for 1 day. She is on irregular follow-up for diabetes management. Husband gives a history of spontaneous miscarriage 5 days before the present visit to the hospital, following 7 weeks of amenorrhea. Clinically, she looks grossly dehydrated, heart rate 124/min, blood pressure 90/46 mmHg with deep laboured breathing at a rate of 28/min. She is dull but arousable and following simple command without any meningeal sign or focal neurological deficit. Arterial blood gas showed: pH 6.79, $PaCO_2$ 6.8 mmHg, $PaO_2$ 82 mmHg (in room air), $HCO_3^-$ 4.8 mmol/L and lactate 2.7 mmol/L. Her capillary blood glucose is 315 mg/dl. Lab results revealed serum $Na^+$—132 mmol/L, serum $K^+$—3.7 mmol/L, serum $Cl^-$—79 mmol/L and urine ketones 3+.



S. Ghosh, *Handbook of Intravenous Fluids*,
https://doi.org/10.1007/978-981-19-0500-1_16

### *16.1.1 What Are the Most Important Steps in Managing Diabetic Ketoacidosis?*

Diabetic ketoacidosis (DKA) is a potentially life-threatening medical emergency usually seen in Type 1 diabetics and occasionally also in Type 2 diabetics. DKA is produced by relative or absolute deficiency of insulin with a relative increase in counterregulatory hormones, which result in hyperglycaemia, osmotic diuresis induced dehydration and electrolyte deficiency, hyperketonaemia and high anion gap metabolic acidosis. It is often precipitated by serious underlying infection or irregular insulin treatment and also due to other stressful conditions like trauma, myocardial infarction etc. Keys to successful management of this condition are timely diagnosis and expeditious management with fluids, electrolyte replacement, insulin administration and management of underlying stressors. Hyperglycaemic hyperosmolar state (HHS) is another related hyperglycaemic emergency, more commonly seen in older patients with type 2 diabetes mellitus, characterized by extreme hyperglycaemia, dehydration, dyselectrolytemia and relative absence of ketosis. In this chapter, we shall discuss key aspects of DKA management. Principles of management for HHS are similar to DKA with only minor changes.

## 16.2 Pathogenesis

- As mentioned earlier, underlying defects in DKA are absolute or relative insulin deficiency and increase in secretion of counterregulatory hormones like glucagon, cortisol and catecholamines, resulting in hyperglycaemia, hyperketonaemia and high anion gap metabolic acidosis.
- **Hyperglycaemia:** Hyperglycaemia results from an increase in gluconeogenesis and glycogenolysis with simultaneous decrease in the uptake of glucose in liver, muscles and other tissues. Hyperglycaemia is further exaggerated in the later stage by renal dysfunction.

- Hyperosmolality resulting from hyperglycaemia produces osmotic diuresis, intravascular volume depletion, dehydration of tissues and multiple electrolyte deficiency including deficiency of whole-body potassium, magnesium and phosphate.
- Hyperglycaemia is known to lower serum sodium levels by drawing intracellular water to the extracellular compartment. In the presence of hyperglycaemia, sodium value should be corrected by adding 1.6 mEq/L for every 100 mg/dL increase in glucose concentration above the level of 100 mg/dl.

- **Hyperketonaemia:** Insulin deficiency, coupled with excess catecholamines, promotes lipolysis, production of increased free fatty acids and triglycerides. In the presence of high counterregulatory hormones especially glucagon, oxidation of free fatty acid is impaired, promoting the production of ketone bodies like acetoacetate and beta-hydroxybutyrate.
  - Resulting hyperketonaemia is further exaggerated by decreased hepatic utilization of ketones.
- **High Anion-Gap (AG) Metabolic Acidosis**: High AG metabolic acidosis results from excessive ketoacid generation that overwhelms both extracellular and intracellular buffering capacity.
  - Apart from high AG metabolic acidosis DKA may also result in other acid-base disorders like normal AG metabolic acidosis from excess 0.9% saline infusion, high AG or normal AG metabolic acidosis from renal dysfunction, metabolic alkalosis from profound vomiting and respiratory alkalosis from hyperventilation.
- Figure 16.1 below summarizes the pathophysiology of DKA.
- **Euglycemic DKA:** Although hyperglycaemia is considered the hallmark of DKA, but in some patients glucose levels may not be that elevated and may remain below 250 mg/dl. This condition is known as euglycemic diabetic ketoacido-

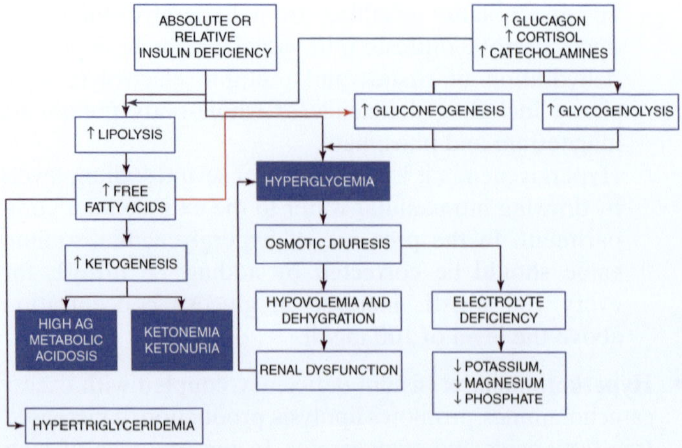


FIGURE 16.1 Pathophysiology of diabetic ketoacidosis

sis and is sometimes seen in patients treated with sodium-glucose co-transporter 2 (SGLT2) inhibitors like canagliflozin, dapagliflozin and empagliflozin. There are three possible explanations for euglycemic diabetic ketoacidosis in patients treated with SGLT-2 inhibitors.

- Lowered insulin dose resulting from the co-prescription of SGLT-2 inhibitors may not be sufficient to suppress lipolysis and ketogenesis.
- Inhibition of SGLT-2 expressed in pancreatic α-cells, promotes glucagon secretion.
- SGLT-2 inhibition may also decrease urinary excretion of ketone bodies.

## 16.3 Diagnosis

- Diabetic ketoacidosis is clinically suspected in the presence of hyperglycaemia with or without polyuria and polydipsia, profound dehydration and metabolic acidosis. DKA may be the initial presentation in some patients with Type 1 DM.

- Kussmaul Breathing may be seen in some patients.
- Hyperketonaemia may manifest with nausea, vomiting, anorexia and abdominal pain.
- An astute clinician may notice the typical fruity-smelling ketonemic breath sometimes.

• Diagnosis is confirmed in the presence of high serum or urine ketone level.

  - Traditional urine dipstick or serum ketone levels using nitroprusside assay cannot detect Beta-hydroxybutyrate, potentially underestimating the severity of the disease at presentation (and over-estimating the same in recovering patients).
  - More recently point-of-care testing of blood ketone levels has been introduced utilizing capillary blood.

• Commonly accepted criteria for the diagnosis of DKA are: blood glucose >250 mg/dl, arterial pH < 7.3, serum $HCO_3^-$ <15 mEq/l and presence of hyperketonaemia or hyperketonuria.
• Apart from confirming the diagnosis, laboratory investigations should focus on measures to monitor disease course and also to look for precipitating factors.

  - Electrolyte abnormalities are common in patients with DKA. They may present initially with hypokalaemia due to low total body potassium levels. However, some patients may have hyperkalaemia because of renal dysfunction or due to impaired movement of potassium from extracellular to intracellular compartment in the presence of metabolic acidosis. Both hypomagnesemia and hypophosphatemia are common requiring correction.
  - It may be a good idea to maintain a chart to follow the progress of the disease. One suggested one is provided in Table 16.1.
  - Hyperamylasaemia may be seen in patients with DKA. In patients of DKA presenting with pain abdomen, it may be prudent to order more specific biochemical tests like lipase or even contrast-enhanced CT abdomen, when acute pancreatitis is strongly suspected.

- Precipitating factors may not be identified in over 50% of cases and in another 30%, DKA is precipitated by noncompliance with insulin therapy. In 12% of patients, there may be some infections especially urinary tract infection and pneumonia. Every effort should be made to look for any underlying infection. DKA can be precipitated by any inter-current medical or stress, e.g. myocardial infarction, stroke, trauma or surgery, prompting appropriate tests.

## 16.4 Management of DKA

- Three most important aspects of DKA management are intravenous fluid therapy, replacement of electrolytes and insulin therapy.
  - It is also equally important to manage any treatable underlying precipitating factors to prevent the recurrence of DKA.
- Patients should be monitored closely throughout the treatment period looking to achieve these above goals without causing any iatrogenic complications.
  - Following parameters should be charted meticulously (as mentioned in Table 16.1): volume status of the patient including input and output, neurological status, serum electrolytes, anion gap, osmolality and glucose.

## 16.5 Fluid Management

- Volume deficits in patients with DKA can be as high as 10–15% of body weight and restoration of both intravascular (and whole body) volume is the key to successful management of DKA. In fact, rehydration itself improves hyperglycaemia independent of insulin administration.
  - Mechanisms for reduction in blood glucose levels following fluid therapy are reduction in counterregulatory

TABLE 16.1 Suggested clinical chart to follow progress of patients with diabetic ketoacidosis

| | **Hour-1** | **Hour-2** | **Hour-3** | **Hour-4** | **Hour-5** | **Hour-6** |
|---|---|---|---|---|---|---|
| *Clinical parameters* | | | | | | |
| Glasgow coma scale | | | | | | |
| Heart rate (/min) | | | | | | |
| MAP (in mmHg) | | | | | | |
| Respiratory rate (/min) | | | | | | |
| Capillary refill time (in second) | | | | | | |
| Total intake (in ml) | | | | | | |
| Total output (in ml) | | | | | | |
| *Biochemical parameters* | | | | | | |
| Blood glucose (in mg/dl) | | | | | | |
| Serum $Na^+$ (in mmol/L) | | | | | | |
| Serum $K^+$ (in mmol/L) | | | | | | |
| Serum $cl^-$ (in mmol/L) | | | | | | |
| Serum $HCO_3^-$ (in mmol/L) | | | | | | |
| Anion gap | | | | | | |
| Ketonuria | | | | | | |
| Ketonemia | | | | | | |

hormones following intravascular volume repletion and effect of haemodilution.

- Intravascular volume repletion should be started before administration of Insulin to avoid worsening of hypovolemia. Insulin infusion facilitates the movement of glucose to the intracellular compartment dragging water along and thus reducing the intravascular volume further.

### *16.5.1 Which Fluid?*

- Isotonic crystalloids are clearly the initial fluid of choice and 0.9% Saline is recommended by the guideline for this purpose [1]. However, in recent years there is a growing concern regarding 0.9% Saline especially in conditions like DKA where large volume of fluid is administered.
  - Large volume of saline administration is associated with hyperchloremia and non-anion gap metabolic acidosis potentially delaying the resolution of DKA. Saline may also be associated with higher risk of renal injury and the association may be dose-dependent.
  - Many experts now believe that balanced salt solutions should be the preferred fluid as they may shorten the time to DKA resolution. However, there are potential issues related to balanced salt solution too, which include risk of increasing cerebral oedema (as balanced solutions are relatively hypotonic) or acetate in Plasmalyte and Sterofundin getting converted to acetoacetate potentially worsening hyperketonemic state.
  - Table 16.2 summarizes clinical studies comparing 0.9% Saline and balanced salt solutions in DKA management.
- Some authors suggested using 0.45% Saline as the choice of fluid if the corrected serum sodium level remains high or normal after initial correction of intravascular volume [9].

Table 16.2 Published studies comparing 0.9% saline and balanced salt solutions in patients with diabetic ketoacidosis

| First author | Type of study | Control | Intervention | Outcome |
|---|---|---|---|---|
| Mahler SA et al. [2] | Single centre.<br>RCT.<br>Adult patients.<br>N = 45 | 0.9% saline | Plasmalyte-A | • Higher bicarbonate and lower chloride at the end of resuscitation in Plasmalyte group.<br>• No difference in patient-centric outcome. |
| Chua HR et al. [3] | Multicentre.<br>Retrospective.<br>Adult patients.<br>N = 23 | 0.9% saline.<br>(N = 14) | Plasmalyte-148.<br>(N = 9) | • Faster resolution of acidosis in Plasmalyte group.<br>• Higher chloride in saline group.<br>• No difference in glycaemic control or ICU-LOS. |
| Van Zyl DG et al. [4] | Single centre. RCT.<br>Adult patients.<br>N = 57 | 0.9% saline | Ringer's lactate | • No statistically significant difference in time to normalization of pH or resolution of DKA between groups. |
| Yung M et al. [5] | Single centre.<br>RCT.<br>Children.<br>N = 77 | 0.9% saline | Hartmann's solution | • No significant difference in time to reach bicarbonate 15 mmol/L or normalization of pH in overall group.<br>• Shorter time for both endpoints with RL in severe subgroup.<br>• No difference in time to SC insulin.<br>• RL group received significantly less total fluid. |

(continued)

Table 16.2 (continued)

| First author | Type of study | Control | Intervention | Outcome |
|---|---|---|---|---|
| Williams V et al. [6] | Single centre.<br>RCT.<br>66 DKA episodes in 64 children. | 0.9% saline | Plasmalyte-A | • No difference in new or progressive AKI.<br>• Median time to resolution of DKA −14.5 h with Plasmalyte A and 16.0 h with saline (P = 0.47).<br>• No difference in resolution of AKI.<br>• No difference in hospital-LOS. |
| Self WH et al. [7] | Subgroup analysis of DKA patients included in two large RCTs (SALT-ED and SMART studies).<br>Adults.<br>N = 172 | 0.9% saline.<br>(N = 78) | Balanced salt solution.<br>Ringer's lactate or Plasmalyte-A.<br>(N = 94) | • Shorter time to DKA resolution (by 20%) and insulin infusion discontinuation (by 30%) in balanced group.<br>• No difference in in-hospital mortality, MAKE-30 or mechanical ventilation days between groups. |
| Ramanan M et al. [8] | Multicentre.<br>Cluster RCT.<br>Adults.<br>N = 90 | 0.9% saline.<br>(N = 48) | Plasmalyte-148.<br>(N = 42) | • Significantly higher rate of DKA resolution at 24-h in Plasmalyte-148 group (69% versus 36%; odds ratio 4.24 (95% CI 1.68–10.72, p 0.002).<br>• Trend for DKA resolution remains higher at 48-h in Plasmalyte-148 group.<br>• No increase in blood ketone level in Plasmalyte-148 group. |

- Based on the current evidence, following fluids may be recommended during the course of DKA management.

  1. In most patients with diabetic ketoacidosis, balanced crystalloids may be the preferred fluid for initial resuscitation, based on strong physiological rationale against using 0.9% saline, none of the clinical studies showing any harm associated with these solutions and most studies showing quicker resolution of DKA with their use.
  2. However, 0.9% Saline may be considered when cost and availability issues are there or when clinician is not anticipating high volume of fluid infusion.
  3. Once the blood glucose level is below 250 mg/dl, it is advised to use dextrose containing fluid (usually 0.45% Saline PLUS 5% Dextrose if the corrected serum sodium level remains high (or normal) and DNS if serum sodium is low) to facilitate continued insulin infusion without causing hypoglycaemia.
  4. Routine use of maintenance fluid should be avoided. Once the anion gap is within normal range and the patient is able to take orally, patients should be allowed orally.

### *16.5.2 What Should Be the Rate of Infusion?*

- One suggested (but somehow arbitrary) approach to fluid therapy is to administer 1 to 2 L fluid over 1 h initially, if the patient is in hypovolemic shock and 500 mL/h for 4 h in other patients, followed by an infusion of 250 mL/h for 4 h and then on as required basis [1, 9].
- There is some concern regarding precipitating cerebral oedema with higher fluid infusion especially in children. However, this concern was refuted convincingly in recent studies [10, 11].
- Following approach is recommended to guide fluid therapy in DKA.

  – Patient should be evaluated for any evidence of circulatory shock. Since shock state must be corrected rapidly,

initial fluid boluses of isotonic crystalloids are advisable. A prudent approach is to administer 500 ml increments of fluids up to a maximum of 15–20 ml/kg body weight over the first 1 h.
- Subsequent fluid boluses should be guided by persistent evidence of shock and fluid responsiveness status of the patient. In the absence of any sophisticated measurements, one approach may be to administer 4 ml/kg boluses of isotonic crystalloids and look for response to the bolus.
- Advanced hemodynamic monitoring should be utilized in patients with underlying renal and cardiac dysfunction.
- No clear guidance can be provided in patients without circulatory shock. One approach can be to continue with daily maintenance fluid infusion till patient is able to take orally plus replacement of volume lost.

## 16.6 Electrolyte Correction

- **Potassium:** Typically in patients with DKA, whole-body potassium deficit ranges from anything between 2 and 5 mEq/kg. As mentioned earlier, this deficit may not be reflected by the serum value of potassium.
  - Insulin administration without correcting hypokalaemia can lower the serum potassium further. Unfortunately, an appropriate strategy for potassium replacement has not been tested in any randomized trial.
  - Initial potassium replacement may be guided by potassium value in arterial blood gas report, pending laboratory measurement. If the potassium level is <3.3 mEq/L, potassium replacement should be initiated urgently at a rate of 40 mEq/litre/h to avoid life-threatening arrhythmias, till potassium reaches 3.3 mEq/L. Till then, insulin administration should be avoided [1, 9].

  - With serum potassium >5.0 or 5.5 mmol/L, potassium supplementation should be avoided till potassium level falls below that value [1, 9].
  - In patients with potassium value between 3.3 to 5 mEq/L and once diuresis is clearly established, potassium supplementation should be started by adding 10 to 40 mmol of potassium in every litre of intravenous fluid [1].

- **Phosphate:** Whole-body phosphate is depleted in DKA. However, randomized studies have failed to confirm any beneficial effect of routine phosphate replacement in clinical outcomes [12]. Moreover, one should keep in mind possibility of intravenous phosphate replacement precipitating hypocalcaemia, especially in patients with borderline or low serum calcium [12].
  - Phosphate replacement is indicated in patients with cardiac dysfunction, severe anaemia, respiratory depression and severe hypophosphatemia (serum phosphate level < 1 mg/dl).
  - 20–30 mEq/l potassium phosphate can be added to replacement fluids. Maximal safe rate of phosphate replacement is 4.5 mEq/h [1].

- **Magnesium:** Hypomagnesemia is common in DKA.
  - Magnesium replacement should be considered in patients with severe hypomagnesemia (serum magnesium <1.2 mg/dl) or in symptomatic patients with cardiac arrhythmias, tremors, paraesthesia, muscle spasms, etc.

- **Bicarbonate**: Severe metabolic acidosis is associated with myocardial dysfunction. However, treating DKA patients routinely with bicarbonate may be counterproductive, as it may precipitate hypokalaemia, potentially delay oxygen uptake at mitochondrial level, worsen cerebral oedema and lead to delayed metabolic alkalosis.
  - One randomized trial has failed to show any clinical benefit of bicarbonate replacement in patients with pH between 6.9 and 7.14 [13].

- However, if the pH is below 6.9, consideration should be given to administering 50 mmol Bicarbonate diluted in 200 ml of 5% Dextrose as 1-h infusion [9].

## 16.7 Insulin

- Insulin should be administered as an intravenous bolus of 0.1 unit/kg, once serum potassium is >3.3 mEq/L and after the administration of initial fluid bolus. An infusion should be started after the initial bolus at a rate of 0.1 unit/kg/h. Blood glucose should be monitored initially on an hourly basis.
  - **Blood Glucose ≥ 250 mg/dl:** Optimal rate of blood glucose reduction is between 50 and 70 mg/dl and insulin dose should be adjusted accordingly.
  - **Blood Glucose < 250 mg/dl:** Infusion rate should be halved once the blood glucose level is below 250 mg/dl. As discussed earlier, some dextrose-containing fluid should be started simultaneously to avoid hypoglycaemia.

    Rate of insulin infusion should be adjusted to keep the blood glucose value between 150 and 200 mg/dl [9].

    Insulin infusion should never be discontinued until complete resolution of DKA.

- Consider switching to subcutaneous insulin once the patient is able to take orally and ketoacidosis is resolved. Criteria for resolution of ketoacidosis are: blood glucose <200 mg/dl and two of the following criteria are fulfilled—serum bicarbonate >15 mEq/l or venous pH >7.3 or calculated anion gap <12 mEq/l [9].
  - To avoid recurrence of DKA, intravenous insulin should be continued for at least 1–2 h after the first dose of subcutaneous insulin.

## 16.8 Case Scenario (Continued)

- Diagnosis of DKA is clear in Mrs. AG. She also shows evidence of hypovolemic shock requiring a litre of intravenous Ringer's lactate in the next 1 h. Further fluid boluses should be guided by evidence of fluid responsiveness.
  - Maintenance fluid infusion containing 20 mEq Potassium per litre of fluid should be commenced after the initial fluid bolus at a rate of approximately 100 ml/h.
  - Insulin infusion should be started after the initial bolus.
  - Consider 50 mmol of bicarbonate as the pH is <6.9.
  - Consider sending serum phosphate and magnesium level and replace them if necessary.

**Take-Home Messages**
- Figure 16.2 summarizes important aspects of managing a patient with DKA.

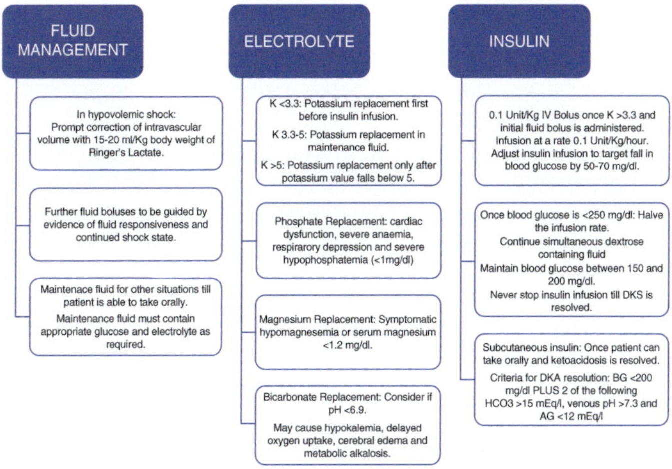


FIGURE 16.2 Management of diabetic ketoacidosis

## References


1. Diabetes Canada Clinical Practice Guidelines Expert Committee, Goguen J, Gilbert J. Hyperglycaemic emergencies in adults. Can J Diabetes. 2018;42 Suppl 1:S109–14.
2. Mahler SA, Conrad SA, Wang H, Arnold TC. Resuscitation with balanced electrolyte solution prevents hyperchloremic metabolic acidosis in patients with diabetic ketoacidosis. Am J Emerg Med. 2011;29:670–4.
3. Chua HR, Venkatesh B, Stachowski E, Schneider AG, Perkins K, Ladanyi S, Kruger P, Bellomo R. Plasmalyte 148 vs 0.9% saline for fluid resuscitation in diabetic ketoacidosis. J Crit Care. 2012;27:138–45.
4. Van Zyl DG, Rheeder P, Delport E. Fluid management in diabetic-acidosis—Ringer's lactate versus normal saline: a randomized controlled trial. QJM. 2012;105:337–43.
5. Yung M, Letton G, Keeley S. Controlled trial of Hartmann's solution versus 0.9% saline for diabetic ketoacidosis. J Paediatr Child Health. 2017;53:12–7.
6. Williams V, Jayashree M, Nallasamy K, Dayal D, Rawat A. 0.9% saline versus plasmalyte as initial fluid in children with diabetic ketoacidosis (SPinK trial): a double-blind randomized controlled trial. Crit Care. 2020;24:1.
7. Self WH, Evans CS, Jenkins CA, Brown RM, Casey JD, Collins SP, et al. Clinical effects of balanced crystalloids vs saline in adults with diabetic ketoacidosis: a subgroup analysis of cluster randomized clinical trials. JAMA Netw Open. 2020;3(11):e2024596.
8. Ramanan M, Attokaran A, Murray L, Bhadange N, Stewart D, Rajendran G, et al. Sodium chloride or plasmalyte-148 evaluation in severe diabetic ketoacidosis (SCOPE-DKA): a cluster, crossover, randomized, controlled trial. Intensive Care Med. 2021;47:1248–57.
9. Kitabchi AE, Umpierrez GE, Miles JM, Fisher JN. Hyperglycaemic crises in adult patients with diabetes. Diabetes Care. 2009;32:1335–43.
10. Kuppermann N, Ghetti S, Schunk JE, Stoner MJ, Rewers A, McManemy JK, et al. Clinical trial of fluid infusion rates for pediatric diabetic ketoacidosis. N Engl J Med. 2018;378:2275–87.

11. Pruitt LG, Jones G, Musso M, Volz E, Zitek T. Intravenous fluid bolus rates and pediatric diabetic ketoacidosis resolution. Am J Emerg Med. 2019;37:2239–41.
12. Fisher JN, Kitabchi AE. A randomized study of phosphate therapy in the treatment of diabetic ketoacidosis. J Clin Endocrinol Metab. 1983;57:177–80.
13. Morris LR, Murphy MB, Kitabchi AE. Bicarbonate therapy in severe diabetic ketoacidosis. Ann Intern Med. 1986;105:836–40.

# Chapter 17
# Disorders of Sodium Balance

## 17.1 Case Scenario 1

Mr. AK, a 44-year-old gentleman, with no known co-morbidities, is admitted with a history of some alteration in his sensorium for the past 1 week. On examination, he is of thin built, weighing about 50 kg. He is dull, lethargic but responding to simple commands. His gums and lips are pigmented (as seen in Fig. 17.1). He has a heart rate of 100/min and blood pressure of 90/50 mmHg. Relevant laboratory findings are Hb—11.4 gm/dl, total count—11,200/mm$^3$ (Eosinophils—21%), serum $Na^+$—106 mmol/L, serum $K^+$—4.9 mmol/L, urine $Na^+$—39 mmol/L, random cortisol—0.74 mcg/dl and normal TSH.

## 17.2 Case Scenario 2

Mrs. AG, a 51-year-old lady was admitted in the floor following abdominal surgery. She underwent laparotomy for ileal perforation. She has been nil per os since the night before surgery and kept on maintenance fluid since surgery with a plan to start oral fluid on postoperative day 4. Her regular medication includes lithium prescribed for bipolar disorder. She is of average built, weighing approximately 60 kg. On



S. Ghosh, *Handbook of Intravenous Fluids*,
https://doi.org/10.1007/978-981-19-0500-1_17

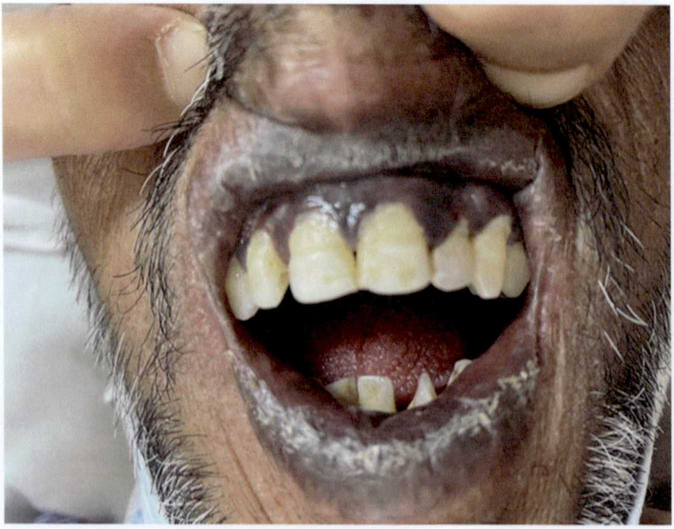

FIGURE 17.1 Pigmented gums and lips

postoperative day 2, she is now unresponsive. Perioperative input is 6250 ml (received only Plasmalyte with $Na^+$ concentration of 140 mmol/L) and urine output is 5870 ml. His current serum $Na^+$ is 168 mmol/L.

## 17.2.1 What are the Most Appropriate Ways to Manage Abnormalities of Serum Sodium?

Disorders of serum sodium are common in acutely ill patients. Unlike disorders of serum potassium, magnesium and calcium, low (hypo-) or high (hyper-) values of serum sodium may not necessarily reflect low or high total body sodium. In fact, hypo- and hypernatremia reflect only the relative concentration of "exchangeable cations" (i.e. $Na^+$ and $K^+$) with total body water [1]. Thus, hyponatremia actually means relative access to water. Whereas hypernatremia reflects a relative deficiency of water. Clinical manifestations of hypo- and hypernatremia result from hypo- or hypertonia and effects of tonicity changes on brain cells, besides manifestations of the underlying disorder itself. In this chapter, we shall discuss the management principles of sodium disorders.

## 17.3 Hyponatremia

- Hyponatremia is defined as serum sodium concentration below 135 mmol/L.
- It can be further classified biochemically as mild (serum $Na^+$ 130–135 mmol/L), moderate (serum $Na^+$ 125–129 mmol/L) and profound (serum $Na^+$ <125 mmol/L) [2].
- Clinical manifestations of hyponatremia depend on the rapidity of its onset and brain cell's ability to adapt to the changes in tonicity of extracellular fluid. Based on the speed of onset, hyponatremia can be again classified as either acute (onset within 48 h) or chronic (hyponatremia lasting for >48 h) [2]. If the onset of hyponatremia cannot be established unequivocally, all hyponatremia should be treated as chronic.

### *17.3.1 Pathophysiology*

- Low serum sodium may simply reflect presence of osmotically active compounds (e.g. glucose or mannitol) in the plasma drawing intracellular fluid out of cell ("Hypertonic Hyponatremia") or inability of the older "flame photometry" method to identify true sodium level because of an increase in solid phase of plasma, e.g. hypertriglyceridemia or paraproteinemia or immunoglobulin treatment ("Isotonic Hyponatremia" or "Pseudohyponatremia").
  - Former conditions can be taken care of by using "correction factor", e.g. for every 100 mg/dl increase in blood glucose above the value of 100 mg/dl add 1.6 mmol/L to get "corrected serum sodium" in the presence of hyperglycaemia.

- Or by using more precise "ion specific" electrodes method for a more accurate value of serum sodium in the presence of "Isotonic Hyponatremia".

- In contrast, "true hyponatremia" is always hypotonic, i.e. serum osmolality below 275 mOsmol/kg.
- **Evolution of Hyponatremia:** True hyponatremia is produced either because of excess free water intake (which by far is rare) or more commonly because of poor excretion of free water.

  - **Excess Free Water:** Three most common causes are:

    **Primary Polydipsia**: Commonly seen in patients with psychiatric illness when excessive water intake (sometimes in excess of 1 Litre/h) exceeds the capacity of kidneys to excrete free water.
    **Iatrogenic**: Inappropriate prescription of large volume of hypotonic fluid.
    Absorption of free water from irrigation fluids that do not contain sodium, used following certain procedures, e.g. following transurethral resection of prostate (TURP) or following gynaecological procedures.

  - **Low Renal Excretion of Free Water:** Possible explanations for low free water excretion are:

    **High Level of Anti-diuretic Hormone (ADH):** High ADH value may be appropriate in the presence of absolute hypovolemia or relative hypovolemia (e.g. chronic liver disease or nephrotic syndrome or chronic heart failure) or may be inappropriate in the absence of physiological stimuli i.e. hypovolemia or hypotonicity ("**Syndrome of Inappropriate ADH or SIADH**"). Postoperative state and pain are important causes of high ADH release. With the loss of inhibitory effects of cortisol, ADH release may increase in the presence of hypercortisolism.

**Low Glomerular Filtration Rate:** Either due to acute kidney injury or in the presence of chronic renal failure.

**Low intake of solutes:** Some solutes are freely excreted through glomeruli but poorly re-absorbed from the tubules, prompting mandatory excretion of free water. These solutes are mostly products of protein metabolism, e.g. urea. When solute load (usually 600 to 900 mOsmol per day in an individual on regular diet) is less, body needs to produce less urine volume to excrete the same load. Typical examples of low solute load conditions are beer potomania or in patients with low protein diet.

- In the presence of hypothyroidism and thiazide diuretics, the exact mechanism for the evolution of hyponatremia is not known and perhaps involves multiple mechanisms.
- Figure 17.2 provides an overview of the evolution of hyponatremia in various conditions.

- **Evolution of Clinical Manifestations in Hyponatremia:** Clinical effects of hyponatremia are because of the effects of resulting hypotonicity on brain cells.
  - In cases of acute hyponatremia (that evolved in <48 h) brain cells swell producing cerebral oedema. Extent of neurological manifestations depends on the level of hyponatremia.
  - In subsequent days, brain cells adapt—initially by rapidly losing electrolytes like sodium, potassium and chloride from cells and later on by loss of intracellular organic solutes like large proteins. Adaption generally takes at least 48 h.
  - Complete adaptation leads to normalization of brain cell volume within several days. However, the overall osmolality of brain cells remains low.

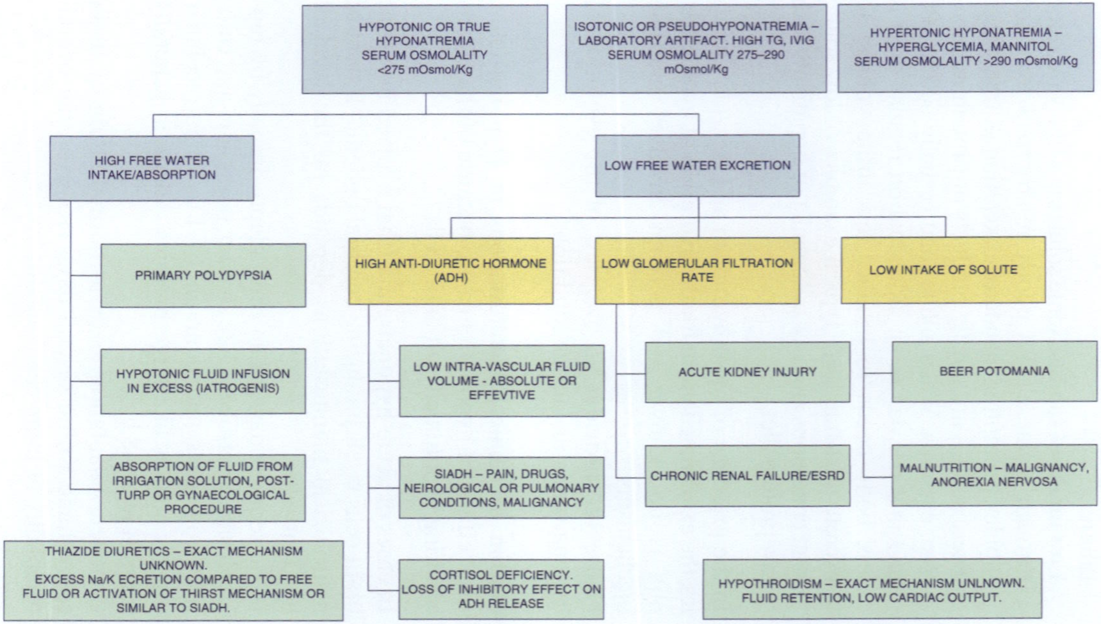


FIGURE 17.2 Evolution of hyponatremia in different conditions

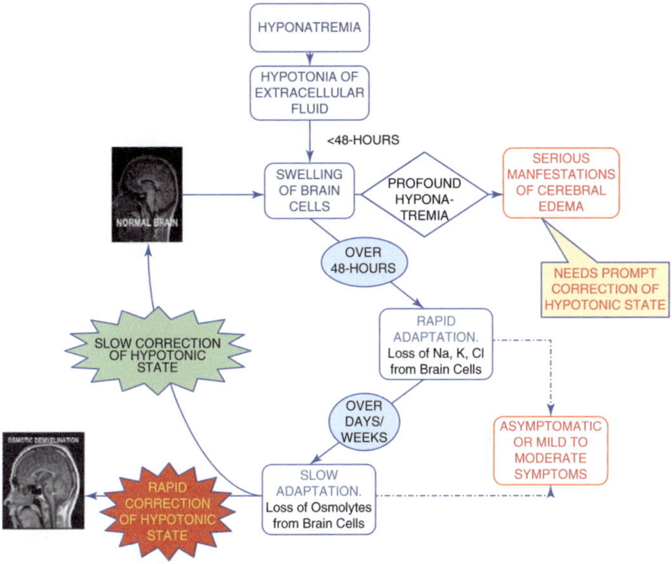


FIGURE 17.3 Hyponatremia, brain cells adaptive responses and consequences of different therapies

- Once brain cells are fully adapted to chronic hyponatraemic state, any aggressive and rapid correction of the hyponatremia may lead to irreversible damage to myelin sheath surrounding brain cells, which leads to a condition called "**Osmotic Demyelination Syndrome (ODS)**".
- Figure 17.3 provides a schematic diaphragm showing the evolution of clinical manifestations of hyponatremia.

## 17.3.2 Clinical Manifestations

- As discussed in the previous section, symptoms of hyponatremia depend both on speed of onset and degree of hyponatremia. Symptoms of hyponatremia are non-specific and may not be explained fully by hyponatremia alone especially when hyponatremia is only of mild or moderate

TABLE 17.1 Symptoms of hyponatremia

| Mild to moderate symptoms | Severe symptoms |
|---|---|
| • Nausea<br>• Some degree of confusion<br>• Headache<br>• Muscle cramps<br>• Lethargy | • Vomiting<br>• Cardiopulmonary distress<br>• Abnormal and deep somnolence<br>• Seizures<br>• Loss of reflexes<br>• Coma |

severity. But with more profound degree of hyponatremia, it is more likely that the symptoms are because of hyponatremia itself.

- Based on symptoms, hyponatremia can be classified as mild to moderate and severe hyponatremia. Symptoms of hyponatremia are shown in Table 17.1 [2].
- Urgency of hyponatremia correction is based on severity of symptoms and the speed or rapidity of its onset and not simply on the degree of hyponatremia.

### 17.3.3 *Diagnostic Approach to Hyponatremia*

- **Step 1:** History and Physical Examination.
  - Apart from symptomatology, history should focus on underlying condition and any prior serum sodium report available to judge the acuteness of symptoms. Acute onset severe symptoms should call for a prompt treatment.
  - Detail medication history including all prescription or non-prescription drugs especially thiazides or common agents responsible for SIADH, e.g. tricyclic antidepressants, carbamazepine, vincristine, chlorpropamide, etc.
  - Any procedures, e.g. postoperative status, history of undergoing TURP, etc.
  - Any underlying neurological or pulmonary conditions that may cause SIADH.
  - Any history suggestive of hypothyroidism or hypocortisolism.

- **Step 2:** Look for Plasma Osmolality.
  - To confirm diagnosis of hypotonic hyponatremia. If it is hypotonic hyponatremia go to Step 3.
  - If plasma osmolality measurement is not readily available, effort should be made to rule out possible causes of hypertonic or isotonic hyponatremia.
- **Step 3:** Send urine osmolality.
  - Urine osmolality <100 mOsmol/kg: Maximal diluting ability of urine is preserved and the cause of hyponatremia is excess free water intake or absorption.
  - Urine osmolality >100 mOsmol/kg: Possible cause of hyponatremia is related to low renal excretion of free water. This can be evaluated further from urine sodium value. Urine sample must be sent simultaneously with blood sample (Go to Step 4).
- **Step 4:** Interpret Urine Sodium Value.
  - Urine Sodium <30 mmol/L: Suggests low effective intravascular volume as the cause of hyponatremia.
  - Urine Sodium >30 mmol/L: Either renal loss of salt (e.g. diuretics or renal salt-wasting nephropathies or cerebral salt-wasting syndrome) or excessive ADH (SIADH or Cortisol deficiency).
- **Step 5:** Check the extravascular volume status.
  - High extracellular fluid (ECF) volume plus low urine sodium: Low effective intravascular volume like CHF or CLD or Nephrotic Syndrome.
  - Low ECF volume plus low urine sodium: True hypovolemic state due to non-renal causes. Example diarrhoea or vomiting.
  - Low ECF volume with high urine sodium: Renal sodium and water loss (sodium loss >> water loss). Example diuretics, salt-losing nephropathies, cerebral salt wasting.

- Normal ECF volume with high urine sodium: SIADH or cortisol deficiency. Hypothyroidism or remote use of diuretic should be ruled out.

- **Step 6:** Specific tests to diagnose specific conditions.
  - Serum Thyroid-Stimulating Hormone, Serum cortisol
  - Renal or liver function tests
  - Imaging: Brain, Lungs

### 17.3.4 *Syndrome of Inappropriate Anti-Diuretic Hormone (SIADH)*

- Diagnosis of SIADH should be made in the presence of all essential criteria given below: [2].
  - Effective serum osmolality <275 mOsm/kg
  - Urine osmolality >100 mOsm/kg
  - Clinical euvolemia
  - Urine Sodium >30 mmol/L with normal dietary salt and water intake
  - Absence of adrenal or thyroid insufficiency
  - No recent use of diuretic agents

### 17.3.5 *Management of Hyponatremia*

- Treatment of hyponatremia is always a balancing act between correcting the risk of cerebral oedema and the risk of osmotic demyelination by overcorrecting the same. The decision is based on severity and duration of symptoms, degree of hyponatremia and volume status of the patient.
  - Hypertonic saline (e.g. 3% Sodium Chloride) should be used only in symptomatic patients.
  - Selective V2-Receptor antagonists (e.g. Tolvaptan, Conivaptan) are no longer recommended for the treatment of hyponatremia [2].

  - One must not forget to initiate cause-specific treatment once the underlying aetiology is clearly established [2].

- Like any other emergency situations priority is to take care of airway, breathing and circulation.
  - Hypovolemia should be corrected rapidly with infusion of 0.9% Saline.

### 17.3.6 Acute Hyponatremia with Severe Symptoms

- **Goal:** To increase the serum sodium level by 5 mmol/L over 1 h. Aim is to promptly reverse symptoms of cerebral oedema.
- **Treatment:** Infuse 2 ml/kg or 100 ml of 3% Saline over 20 min. 3% Saline bolus may be repeated up to two more times, if severe symptoms persist [2, 3].
- **Monitor:** Improvement in symptoms. Repeat serum sodium after 1-h. If the patient remains symptomatic even after an increase in serum sodium by 5 mmol/L or after 3 boluses of 3% saline, other diagnostic possibilities should be explored.
- **Further Management:** If the patient improves with these measures, continue with 3% saline infusion.
  - Set a revised goal of limiting the increase in serum sodium value to a total of 10 mmol/L in the first 24 h and an additional 8 mmol/L during every subsequent 24 h till serum sodium value reaches not more than 130 mmol/L.
  - Monitor serum sodium at regular intervals—every 6 or 8 h for the first 24 h and then at least once a day and readjust the rate of 3% Saline infusion accordingly.

### *17.3.7 Chronic Hyponatremia with Mild to Moderate Symptoms*

- **Goal:** To increase serum sodium value to a total of 10 mmol/L in the first 24 h and an additional 8 mmol/L during every subsequent 24 h, till serum sodium value reaches 130 mmol/L.
- **Treatment:** 3% Saline infusion. Dose of 3% Saline is calculated using Adrogué and Madias formula [4].
  - 1000 ml of 3% Saline infusion is expected to change serum Sodium concentration (in mmol/L) by:

$$\frac{\text{Infusate Sodium}(\text{in mmol / L}) - \text{Serum Sodium}(\text{in mmol / L})}{\text{Total Body Water}(\text{in Litre}) + 1}$$

  - Sodium concentration in 3% Saline: 513 mmol/L.
  - Total body water: 60% of body weight for a young male and 50% of body weight for a young female. The values are 50% and 45% respectively for elderly males and females.
  - Example: For a young man weighing 70 kg and current serum sodium value of 110 mmol/L, expected change in serum sodium following 1000 ml 3% Saline infusion, is approximately 9.37 mmol ([513 – 110] ÷ [70 × 0.6 + 1]). Hence, for 10 mmol/L change in serum sodium over 24 h 1067 ml of 3% saline needs to be infused over 24-h, at a rate of approximately 45 ml/h.

- **Monitor:** In reality change in serum sodium may not follow the expected rule and serum sodium needs to be monitored at regular intervals—initially every 6 or 8 h for the first 24-h and then at least once a day and readjust infusion rate of 3% Saline.

  - Change in serum potassium level also influences change in sodium (as it influences total exchangeable ions) [1].

- Sudden increase in urine volume up to >100 ml/h suggests suppression of ADH (because of hypovolemia correction). This should prompt clinician to go for a more frequent monitoring of sodium concentration [2].

### 17.3.8 Chronic Hyponatremia with Severe Hyponatremia

- No general recommendation can be made for this scenario. Clinician should weigh the risk of cerebral oedema with the risk of ODS.
- It is perhaps advisable to treat patients with the most severe symptoms like coma or seizure with more rapid correction of sodium, as discussed above in the section on acute hyponatremia with severe symptoms.
- Other patients can be treated as chronic hyponatremia with mild to moderate symptoms.

### 17.3.9 Asymptomatic Hyponatremia

- 3% Saline infusion should be avoided in patients with asymptomatic hyponatremia.
- Focus should be to correct volume status of the patients.
  - Hypovolemia should be treated with infusion of 0.9% Saline.
  - Patients with extracellular fluid accumulation and hyponatremia should be treated with salt and fluid restriction and judicious use of loop diuretics. Underlying conditions need to be treated appropriately.
  - Fluid restriction to less than 1-Litre/day should be the initial treatment option for euvolemic patients with hyponatremia (SIADH, cortisol deficiency) who are otherwise asymptomatic. Guidelines suggest, oral urea at a dose of 0.25–0.50 g/kg urea as an additional treatment option aiming for an increased solute intake [2].

### *17.3.10 Osmotic Demyelination Syndrome (ODS)*

- ODS occurs as a result of rapid correction of chronic hypotonic state and is most commonly seen following rapid correction of serum sodium in a patient with chronic hyponatremia [5]. Certain subgroup of patients is particularly at a risk of ODS e.g. malnutrition, chronic alcoholism, associated profound hypokalaemia, liver disease [5].
- Clinical manifestations of ODS are related to particular area of brain involved. Based on particular area of the brain involved, ODS is classified into two groups: Central Pontine Myelinolysis (CPM, involvement of pons) and Extrapontine Myelinolysis (EPM, involvement of basal ganglia, hippocampus, thalamus, cerebellum, central cortex).
  - Manifestations of CPM include dysarthria, dysphagia, quadriplegia (initially flaccid, later on spastic) and classic "locked-in syndrome".
  - EPM produces delayed movement disorders including dystonia, catatonia and Parkinsonism.
- There is no specific treatment for ODS. Hence it is important to avoid too rapid correction of chronic hyponatremia.
  - Guideline recommends re-lowering of serum sodium, if total increase in sodium concentration exceeds the recommended limit of 10 mmol/L in first 24 h or 8 mmol/L in any 24 h thereafter [2].
  - Guideline further suggests infusion of 5% Dextrose solutions at a rate of 10 ml/kg over 1 h under supervision in case serum sodium increases beyond a recommended limit, in addition to stopping ongoing 3% Saline infusion [2].

## 17.4 Hypernatremia

- Hypernatremia is defined as serum sodium concentration above 145 mmol/L. Compared to hyponatremia, hypernatremia is less common, but it carries a worse prognosis [6].

### 17.4.1 *Pathophysiology*

- Like true hyponatremia, hypernatremia is also produced by abnormalities of body fluid with a relatively higher concentration of exchangeable solutes (mainly sodium but also potassium). Hypernatremia develops either because of the loss of both solute and water with water loss disproportionately more than solute loss or because of pure water loss or (rarely) because of gain of sodium [7].
  - Hypernatremic state is usually compounded by inability to consume enough water—extremes of age, altered mental status or intubated state.
- **Water and solute loss:** Loss of water and solute may be either because of extrarenal loss or because of some disorder of renal concentrating ability.
  - **Extra-renal Mechanism:**

    Excess loss through intact skin, e.g. fever, high ambient temperature, heavy exercise or through non-intact skin e.g. large wound or burn.
    Gastrointestinal Loss, e.g. through fistula, diarrhoeal illnesses, laxative.
  - **Renal Mechanism:**

    Osmotic diuretic, e.g. Mannitol, hyperglycaemic states.
    Loop diuretics.
    High solute intake, e.g. through parenteral nutrition.
    Post-obstructive diuresis or polyuric phase of acute tubular necrosis.
    Intrinsic defect in renal concentrating ability.
- **Loss of pure water:** Diabetes insipidus.
  - Central, e.g. following traumatic brain injury, subarachnoid haemorrhage, meningitis, encephalitis, brain tumours, etc.

  - Nephrogenic, e.g. congenital or acquired (hypercalcemia, hypokalaemia, drugs, e.g. lithium, amphotericin B, demeclocycline).

- **Sodium Gain:**
  - Treatment with Hypertonic saline or Sodium bicarbonate.
  - Improper correction of diabetes insipidus with 0.9% saline.

- Clinical manifestations of hypernatremia are produced by shrinkage of brain cells in the presence of hypertonic state. Hypertonicity may produce extreme shrinkage of brain, leading even to rupture of cerebral vessels, subdural or subarachnoid haemorrhage. Later condition is more commonly seen in elderly patients.

### 17.4.2 *Clinical Manifestations and Diagnosis*

- Clinical features of hypernatremia are due to disturbances of cerebral function. It is more common when the change in serum sodium concentration is large or when the change occurs rapidly or for both reasons.
- Symptoms range from irritability, altered mental status, hyperreflexia to seizure and coma. As mentioned earlier, hypernatremia may lead to intracranial haemorrhage and permanent neurological damage.
- As these patients are critically ill with many of them having underlying brain diseases, sometimes it may be difficult to differentiate symptoms of hypernatremia from that of an underlying condition.
- Simple laboratory tests like blood glucose can establish the diagnosis easily.
- For diagnosing diabetes insipidus, water deprivation test may be performed, provided the patient is stable. Urine osmolality is checked after 8 h of water deprivation.

- Urine osmolality remaining below 300 mOsmol/L despite rise in plasma osmolality establishes the diagnosis of diabetes insipidus in a polyuric patient.
- To differentiate between Central and Nephrogenic Diabetes Insipidus, inject now 5 Units of vasopressin subcutaneously. Rise in urine osmolality above 600 mOsmol/L after 1 h of vasopressin administration confirms presence central diabetes insipidus.

### *17.4.3 Management of Hypernatremia*

- Apart from taking care of airway, breathing and circulation, three important measures to manage hypernatremia are restoration of intravascular volume, treat underlying aetiology and correction of hypertonicity.
- **Restoration of intravascular volume:** In patients with obvious intravascular volume depletion as manifested by dry mucous membrane, shrunken eye, delayed capillary refill time with or without hypotension, priority is to restore intravascular volume quickly. Best fluid option for this purpose is isotonic balanced crystalloids.
- **Treatment of underlying aetiology:**
  - Stop diuretics and laxatives.
  - Treat hyperglycaemia with insulin.
  - Treatment of central diabetes insipidus with desmopressin nasal spray or subcutaneous vasopressin and nephrogenic diabetes insipidus with removal of underlying cause (treat hypercalcemia/hypokalaemia or remove causative drugs like lithium) or thiazide.
- **Correction of Hypertonicity:** Hypertonicity correction must be balanced against the risk of precipitating cerebral oedema. Hence, the correction must be slow—decrease of serum sodium by 0.5 mmol/L/h to a maximum of 10 mmol over 24 h. Serum sodium must be monitored periodically, initially every 6 to 8 h for first 24-h and then at least once every day.

- Preferred fluid of choice is plain water administered orally or enterally, whenever feasible. However, in critically ill patients, hypotonic fluids like 5% Dextrose or 0.45% Saline may be required.
- Total fluid required is calculated by volume required to change serum sodium concentration by a desired level (using Adrogué and Madias formula) PLUS daily maintenance fluid volume [7].
- 1000 ml of hypotonic fluid infusion is expected to change serum Sodium concentration (in mmol/L) by:

$$\frac{\text{Infusate Sodium}(\text{in mmol / L}) - \text{Serum Sodium}(\text{in mmol / L})}{\text{Total Body Water}(\text{in Litre}) + 1}$$

- Total body water: 60% of body weight for a young male and 50% of body weight for a young female. The values are 50% and 45%, respectively, for elderly males and females, respectively.
  - Example: For a 70 kg young male with traumatic brain injury and fever, who has received mannitol and whose current serum sodium concentration is 160 mmol/L, expected fall in serum sodium following 1000 ml 5% Dextrose (with sodium concentration 0 mmol/L), is approximately 3.72 mmol ([0 – 160] ÷ [70 × 0.6 + 1]).
  - Hence, for 10 mmol/L change in serum sodium over 24 h 2688 ml 5% Dextrose is required over 24-h. Maintenance fluid requirement for 24 h is approximately 2500 ml.
  - Total fluid required: 2688 + 2500 = 5188 ml over 24-h.
  - Maintenance fluid requirement can often be delivered orally or enterally.
- In patients with hypokalaemia requiring potassium-containing fluid, modified Adrogué and Madias formula can be used. One thousand millilitre of potassium-containing hypotonic fluid is expected to change serum Sodium concentration (in mmol/L) by [7]:

$$\frac{\left[\text{Infusate Sodium} + \text{Infusate Potassium}\left(\text{in mmol / L}\right)\right] - \text{Serum Sodium}\left(\text{in mmol / L}\right)}{\text{Total Body Water}\left(\text{in Litre}\right) + 1}$$

- In patients with hypernatremia due to sodium gain, loop diuretics should be administered to enhance sodium excretion, in addition to hypotonic fluid infusion [7].

## 17.5 Case Scenario (Continued)

- **Case Scenario 1:** Underlying aetiology of hyponatremia in Mr. AK is hypocortisolism resulting from disseminated tuberculosis, which was confirmed by further investigations. He needs treatment with steroid replacement and anti-tubercular medication.
  - Since he is having mild to moderate symptoms of hyponatremia, it may be worth treating him with 3% Saline infusion. However, the initial target should be lower, considering his underlying malnutrition, maybe 8 mmol/L increase of sodium concentration over the next 24 h.
  - 1000 ml 3% Saline will change the serum sodium by 13.12 mmol/L ([513 − 106] ÷ [50 × 0.6 + 1]). Thus, to change serum sodium by 8 mmol/L, volume of 3% Saline required is 609 ml to be infused over 24 h at a rate of ~25 ml/h.
  - Serum sodium should be monitored periodically at 8-hourly intervals.
- **Case Scenario 2:** Possible cause of hypernatremia in Mrs. AG is possibly Nephrogenic Diabetes Mellitus (with Lithium as the underlying cause) worsened further by isotonic maintenance fluid and lack of access to free water.
  - Hypertonicity can be corrected by 5% Dextrose infusion.
  - Total Body Water: 60 × 0.5 = 30 kg.

- Sodium change by 1 Litre of 5% Dextrose is 5.4 mmol/L, ([0 − 168] ÷ [60 × 0.5 + 1]). Hence, approximately 1850 ml of 5% Dextrose is required for 10 mmol reduction in sodium concentration over 24 h.
- Considering maintenance fluid requirement of approximately 2300 ml, total volume of 5% Dextrose to be transfused over 24 h is 4150 ml at an initial rate of ~170 ml/h.
- Again at least 8-hourly monitoring of serum sodium will be required for making adjustment in infusion rate.

**Take-Home Messages**

- Disorders of serum sodium are determined by the balance between extracellular fluid and exchangeable cations.
- Appropriate management hypo- and hypernatremia should be based on the severity of symptoms, speed of onset of symptoms and underlying disease process.
- Every attempt should be made to diagnose underlying disease process leading to sodium disorders and manage the same.
- Correction of sodium disorders should be done in a measured way to avoid iatrogenic complications.

## References

1. Edelman IS, Leibman J, O'Meara MP, Birkenfeld LW. Interrelations between serum sodium concentration, serum osmolarity and total exchangeable sodium, total exchangeable potassium and total body water. J Clin Invest. 1958;37:1236–56.
2. Spasovski G, Vanholder R, Allolio B, Annane D, Ball S, Bichet D, et al. Clinical practice guideline on diagnosis and treatment of hyponatraemia. Intensive Care Med. 2014;40:320–31.
3. Overgaard-Steensen C, Ring T. Clinical review: practical approach to hyponatraemia and hypernatremia in critically ill patients. Crit Care. 2013;17(1):206.

4. Adrogué HJ, Madias NE. Hyponatremia. N Engl J Med. 2000;342(21):1581–9.
5. Martin RJ. Central pontine and extrapontine myelinolysis: the osmotic demyelination syndromes. J Neurol Neurosurg Psychiatry. 2004;75 Suppl 3(Suppl 3):iii22–8.
6. Stelfox HT, Ahmed SB, Khandwala F, Zygun D, Shahpori R, Laupland K. The epidemiology of intensive care unit-acquired hyponatraemia and hypernatremia in medical-surgical intensive care units. Crit Care. 2008;12(6):R162.
7. Adrogué HJ, Madias NE. Hypernatremia. N Engl J Med. 2000;342:1493–9.

# Part V
# Practical Aspect of Intravenous Fluid Management

# Chapter 18
# Prescription of Intravenous Fluid

*All things are poison and nothing (is) without poison; only the dose makes that a thing is no poison.*

*—Paracelsus*

Fluids are medications and like any other medication prescription of intravenous fluids needs careful consideration of indication, appropriate selection of agent, appropriate dosing and of course the cost involved (both direct and indirect). Like any other medical treatment, fluid therapy also needs to be monitored periodically for desirable effects and any adverse effects. Finally, intravenous fluids also cannot be prescribed for an indefinite period, requiring a decision about the discontinuation of the same at an appropriate time. In this chapter, we shall discuss various aspects of intravenous fluid prescription at the bedside including "right indication", "right fluid", "right dose", "right rate of infusion" and "right duration". An example of a typical intravenous fluid prescription is given in Fig. 18.2 at the end of this chapter.



S. Ghosh, *Handbook of Intravenous Fluids*,
https://doi.org/10.1007/978-981-19-0500-1_18

## 18.1 Right Indication

- Fluid requirements for vast majority of hospitalized patients, especially those who are in the floor or wards, can be fulfilled by oral or enteral route unless the patient is either unable to take anything orally or not allowed oral fluid for therapeutic reasons. Thus, the need for intravenous fluid prescription is limited to a small number of patients, mostly from intensive care units or operating room or emergency room or victims of trauma in the field.
  - Before prescribing intravenous fluid, the prescriber needs to ask him- or herself: "Why does my patient need intravenous fluid".

    Is it to supplement normal fluid requirement or to completely supplant it because the patient's oral intake is limited or enteral route is not available at all?
    Is it to replace fluid lost in excess through gastrointestinal, urinary or cutaneous route, that cannot be replaced solely by oral or enteral route?
    Is it to resuscitate patients with relative (in distributive shock) or absolute hypovolemia?

- Intravenous route is preferred in patients with circulatory shock requiring fluid resuscitation. But in a desperate situation with the non-availability of resources, an attempt should be made to correct hypovolemia in shock patients using enteral route through a nasogastric tube.
  - In an interesting study from France, 50 patients with septic shock were resuscitated either with 500 ml of fluid administered through enteral route over 15 min or 500 ml of 0.9% Saline administered intravenously over 15 min [1].
  - Observed increase in "Stroke Volume" following fluid administration did not differ between groups. Both groups showed significant improvement in blood pressure and peripheral perfusion parameters.
  - However, findings of this study need to be validated in larger cohort(s) including sicker patients.

## 18.2 Right Fluid

- While choosing the right intravenous fluid, the following factors need to be considered:
  - Indication for intravenous fluid therapy
  - Composition of the fluid: Electrolytes content, strong ion difference and tonicity
  - Possible adverse consequences: In a particular patient for whom it is intended to be used
  - Clinical condition of the patient: Renal or hepatic dysfunction or risk of raised intracranial pressure (ICP)
  - Patient's serum electrolyte concentration: Especially serum sodium, potassium and chloride
  - Cost of individual commercially available fluid
- Moderately hypotonic fluid containing dextrose is preferred as maintenance fluid in most adult patients.
  - Example: 0.45% Saline with 5% Dextrose with or without Potassium supplement (based on patient's serum Potassium value). Alternatively, Isolyte-M can be used for the same purpose.
  - However, in patients at a risk of raised ICP, slightly hypertonic fluid with dextrose will be the appropriate maintenance fluid of choice. Example: 5% DNS (not to forget the risk of hyperglycaemia in these patients and possible need to rectify the same).
- The composition of replacement fluid should ideally match the lost fluid content.
  - Example: replacement of chloride-rich gastric fluid (through refractory vomiting) should be either by chloride-rich 0.9% Saline or commercially available Isolyte G.
  - In most patients with diarrheal illness, preferred replacement fluid should be Ringer's Lactate or other buffered Isotonic Solution.
- Appropriate choice of fluid for resuscitation purpose should be warm buffered isotonic solution with the sole

exception of patients at a risk of raised ICP where 0.9% Saline or commercially available Sterofundin should be used.

- In patients with haemorrhagic shock, resuscitation may start with warm isotonic solution cautiously. But as soon as possible, transfusion of Packed Red Blood Cell, Random Donor Platelet and Fresh Frozen Plasma must be initiated at a ratio of 1:1:1 to 1:1:2.

## 18.3 Right Dose

- While prescribing intravenous fluid, dose must be mentioned clearly in the prescription. Not surprisingly, it may not be feasible to decide the dose for the whole day especially during resuscitation.
- Initial dose may be simply:
  - Example 1: Please infuse 500 ml of Lactated Ringer's solution through a peripheral IV access for over 15 min.
  - Example 2: Please infuse 2400 ml of 0.45% Saline with 5% Dextrose solution through a peripheral access over the next 24 h at a rate of 100 ml/h. Please add 20 mEq Potassium in two of the 500 ml bags of IV Fluid.
  - But the prescription should never be in the fashion as depicted in Fig. 18.1.

- Intravenous fluid dosing is a dynamic process requiring constant monitoring for the desired effect, as well as for any adverse consequences. Decision for further fluid dosing should be based on the parameters mentioned below:
  - During resuscitation, tests for fluid responsiveness or fluid challenge should be frequently used to assess the need for further fluid.
  - Patients should be monitored for tissue perfusion parameters like warm peripheries, appropriate mentation, capillary refill time, urine output or lactate.

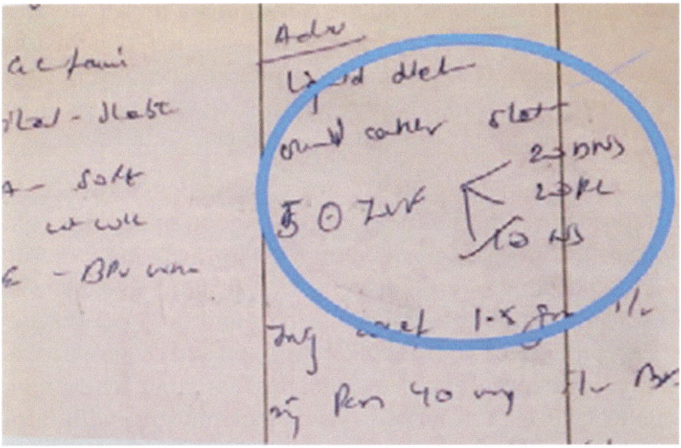

FIGURE 18.1 Wrong prescription of intravenous fluid

- Evidence of worsening low SID (or normal anion gap) metabolic acidosis or pulmonary oedema or worsening intra-abdominal pressure should prompt prescriber to stop further fluid infusion. In cases of worsening metabolic acidosis change in the choice of fluid should be considered.

## 18.4 Right Rate of Infusion

- As explained above, rate of fluid infusion is again dynamic and should be based on response to initial fluid or the need for further fluid. But as explained in examples 1 and 2 above the rate of infusion must be clearly mentioned in the prescription.
  - Peripheral IV Cannulas are preferred for rapid infusion of intravenous fluids as they usually have larger bore (up to 14 or 16 G) and shorter length, compared to central venous catheters. They are also easily accessible to most patients.

- However, in some patients, for example in patients with severe burn injury or in long-stay or oedematous patients in ICU, getting a peripheral access may be difficult. They may require central venous access or in extreme cases even venous cut-down.

- In some difficult patients, a dialysis catheter (especially those with a third lumen) may be a good option for rapid transfusion. Classic example may be in patients requiring blood products during massive transfusion.
- All intravenous access should be monitored periodically for evidence of thrombophlebitis (pain and redness), infection (evidence of redness, pain, pus discharge or fever and leucocytosis), thrombosis (periodic monitoring with ultrasound) or blockage. All precautions should be taken to avoid these complications.

## 18.5 Right Duration

- There should be a plan regarding discontinuation of intravenous fluid at the initiation of the prescription itself.
  - In patients with circulatory shock, enteral (or oral) feeding should be initiated when vasopressors are no longer in escalating dose, peripheral perfusion is significantly restored and the gut is available otherwise. Intravenous fluid can be discontinued once maintenance fluid requirement of the patient can be satisfied with enteral feeding itself [2, 3].
  - Similarly, as soon as possible oral (or enteral) feeding should be started post-abdominal surgery and intravenous maintenance fluid should be stopped [2].

- If the enteral feeding cannot be initiated, because of non-functioning gut or gastrointestinal intolerance, prescription of parenteral nutrition should be considered.
  - Guidelines suggest the initiation of parenteral nutrition if oral or enteral nutrition cannot be initiated in an ICU patient even after 1-week or maybe earlier in selected patients with pre-existing malnutrition [2].

**Take-Home Messages**

- Prescription of intravenous fluid must be individualized and logical considering "Right Indication", "Right Fluid", "Right Rate" and "Right Duration".
- A suggested prescription of intravenous maintenance fluid is provided in Fig. 18.2.
- All patients must be monitored periodically for desired effects of the infusion, as well as for any of its adverse consequences.
- As soon as possible, fluid should be started preferably through oral route or at least enterally. Selected patients may require parenteral route to fulfil their fluid, electrolyte and nutritional requirement for a longer duration.

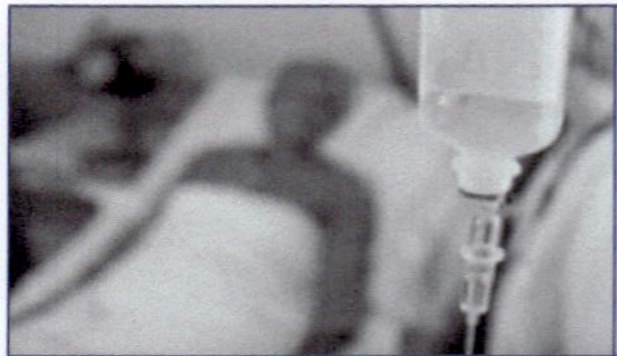

- 58 Years old woman. No co-morbidity. Weight - 70 Kg.
- Admitted to the hospital following jejunal perforation from a diverticular ulcer.
- Underwent resection-anastomosis under General Anesthesia and peritoneal toileting.
- Admitted in the HDU for observation post-surgery. She is hemodynamically stable with nasogastric tube, an abdominal drain and Foley catheter in place.

| | |
|---|---|
| **INDICATION FOR INTRAVENOUS FLUID PRESCRIPTION** | Maintenance fluid in a Post-operative Patient with paralytic ileus |

| FLUID TYPE | VOLUME | ADDITIVE | INFUSION RATE | DURATION | REASSESSMENT |
|---|---|---|---|---|---|
| 0.45% Saline + 5% Dextrose | 2500 ml | 20 ml of 15% Potassium Chloride in First 1000 ml of fluid | 104 ml/ Hour | 24 Hours | 1. Hourly assessment of urine output, output from abdominal drain and nasogastric suction.<br>2. Hourly assessment of peripheral perfusion, heart rate and blood pressure.<br>3. Hourly assessment of respiratory status including respiratory rate and SpO2.<br>4. Monitoring of abdominal pressure if required. |

FIGURE 18.2 Example of an ideal intravenous fluid prescription. $SpO_2$ oxygen saturation by pulse oximetry

# References


1. Guinot PG, Nguyen M, Duclos V, Soudry-Faure A, Bouhemad B, Water Study Group. Oral water ingestion in the treatment of shock patients: a prospective randomized study. Intensive Care Med. 2020;46:2111–2.
2. Taylor BE, McClave SA, Martindale RG, Warren MM, Johnson DR, Braunschweig C, et al. Society of Critical Care Medicine; American Society of Parenteral and Enteral Nutrition. Guidelines for the provision and assessment of nutrition support therapy in the adult critically ill patient: Society of Critical Care Medicine (SCCM) and American Society for Parenteral and Enteral Nutrition (A.S.P.E.N.). Crit Care Med. 2016;44:390–438.
3. Rhodes A, Evans L, Alhazzani W, Levy M, Antonelli M, Ferrer R, et al. Surviving sepsis campaign: international guidelines for management of sepsis and septic shock: 2016. Crit Care Med. 2017;45:486–552.

# Index





S. Ghosh, *Handbook of Intravenous Fluids*,
https://doi.org/10.1007/978-981-19-0500-1

MIX
Papier aus verantwortungsvollen Quellen
Paper from responsible sources
FSC® C105338

If you have any concerns about our products, you can contact us on
**ProductSafety@springernature.com**

In case Publisher is established outside the EU, the EU authorized representative is:
**Springer Nature Customer Service Center GmbH**
**Europaplatz 3, 69115 Heidelberg, Germany**

Printed by Libri Plureos GmbH
in Hamburg, Germany